Hannah's Choice

A daughter's love for life.
The mother who let her make the
hardest decision of all.

HANNAH & KIRSTY JONES

HarperCollinsPublishers

HarperCollins*Publishers*
77–85 Fulham Palace Road,
Hammersmith, London W6 8JB

www.harpercollins.co.uk

First published by HarperCollins*Publishers* 2010

A catalogue record for this book is
available from the British Library

ISBN 978-0-00-734236-5

Find out more about HarperCollins and the environment at
www.harpercollins.co.uk/green

To all the staff on the paediatric ward at
Hereford County Hospital

Contents

CHAPTER ONE

Seize the Moment

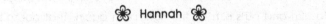 Hannah

So what are the really important things you need to know about me? Well, first there's the fact that if I ever have a boyfriend I want him to look like Zac Efron. At the moment, though, I don't want a boyfriend. My friend Simone has one called Tiago and we've nicknamed them Barbie and Ken. But I'm not interested because I don't want anyone tagging onto me. I've got more important things to do.

Simone is one of my school friends and the others are Laura, Becky, Kelcea, Brigitta and Zoe. They're all nutters and we're always in touch, even though I don't see them much because at the moment I'm not well enough to go to school a lot of the time. When I'm at home, though, they message me to find out how I am or to tell me what's happening because there's usually something going on – like when two of them once stopped speaking and I just wanted to bang their heads together. But I had to wait until I got back to school and by then they'd made up again. Mostly, though, we all get on really well and do girly stuff like trying out makeup on each other or having sleepovers. Once I stayed up until 11 p.m. on a school night and felt like a zombie the next day.

Then there's my family. First off is my dad Andrew, who's forty-three and really big and round so you get better cuddles. Mostly he smiles and is always winding me up by making jokes. But sometimes he blows his top when he gets angry and shouts the house down so we have to leave him alone until Mum speaks to him and puts him on the right path again. That doesn't happen often, though, because he's usually in a good mood. He's a really nice dad.

My mum Kirsty is forty-two. Small with long red hair, she has twinkly eyes and loves horses almost as much as she loves my brother, sisters and I. She's a really good mum and on the days I'm feeling well we'll do things like bake cakes and biscuits. But if I'm feeling tired we'll stay quiet and she'll sometimes even go to the shop to get me juice and magazines. The best thing she did recently, though, was deciding to have a week when we didn't answer the phone. Our house can get really busy some-times and I just wanted it all to slow down because I felt so tired. That was when Mum took the phone off the hook and I really enjoyed it.

Then there are my younger brother and sisters. First comes Oli, who's twelve and will hit you if he's in a bad mood. But if he's in a good one he'll help you get past the really hard levels on your Nintendo DS – sitting there for ages working out how to get past obstacles or putting in cheat codes if he can't – which I really like. Mostly Oli is quiet and shy but he's chatty with me when he wants to be.

Next comes Lucy, who's ten. She's outgoing, always wants to beat everyone to be the best and is almost as horse-mad as Mum. In fact she's so good at show jumping that she's hoping to go to the Olympics some day. She goes away a lot because she competes in shows at weekends and I miss her because I can't go. There's no heating in the horse trailer and I'd get too cold if I did, which isn't good when your heart is bad.

But when Lucy is at home we talk about horses all the time – sitting and looking at pony magazines and deciding which ones we'd buy if we had loads of money – and I love it when I do get to go to shows with her because we eat loads of burgers. I've tried riding myself but I'm scared of heights and have a weak ankle which isn't a good combination to have on a horse.

Finally there's Phoebe, who's four and wild. Mum sometimes says she could swear she was given the wrong baby at hospital because Phoebe will run round the house again and again and never get tired. She goes at fifty miles an hour – banging the lounge doors so you know where she is – which is amazing because when she was born she weighed less than two bags of sugar and now you couldn't miss her. Phoebe also loves riding, but while most girls her age have a leading rein she doesn't have one because she's so brave. She'll always put up a good fight with me but she's kind too and will share her chocolates or give me a one pence piece which she thinks is a lot of money.

Then there are our animals, and there are lots of those. We've got a dog called Ted, a cat called Tails McFluff, some goldfish (although Tails ate some of them once) and ponies called Roxie, Buddy and Mr Minty for Mum, Lucy and Phoebe to ride. We also have chickens for eggs but aren't allowed to play with them because we put one on the trampoline in the garden once and laughed as it bounced up before flying away. Mum really told us off so we knew we couldn't do that again.

Then there's me. I'm thirteen and I don't spend nearly so much time running around as Oli, Lucy and Phoebe because I've got a bad heart and get tired easily. That's why I only go to hospital school in the mornings and then come home at lunchtime to rest. I also spend a lot of time in bed because I pick up any little infection going like colds or stomach upsets which can get really boring because when I feel really ill my energy goes and all I can do is lie quietly.

But when I get well I get busy again, although I call it 'lazy busy' because I can't run around or climb trees. Instead I do stuff like reading, going on my laptop, watching TV or playing DS in my bedroom. I'm lucky because it's my favourite place in the world, all pink with a four-poster bed, and my room at Acorns, where I go once a month, is cool too. Acorns is a place where children who are really ill can have a rest.

The films I like are *Enchanted* and *High School Musical* even though I know it's not cool for someone as old as me to enjoy films like that. So I don't tell my friends, who are all into bands like Evanescence and Paramore, in case they think I'm babyish. But I prefer happy stuff and that's why I like those films and the music in them. On TV I enjoy *Lark Rise to Candleford* and detective programmes like *Poirot* because I try and work out the case before the policeman does. I watch *EastEnders* sometimes too, even though Mum doesn't really like me to, but not that often because the people in Albert Square are always having massive fights so it can get a bit predictable.

I also like *The Apprentice* when Sr'Alan tells the contestants where they're going wrong, and *Strictly Come Dancing*. I love Anton because he smiles so much, and Brendan, who's always going off in a major strop. Bruce Forsyth is really old but good and Tess is nice too, although she sometimes wears odd dresses. I prefer *Strictly* to *The X Factor* because the people don't know if they can dance and some of them get really good while others are awful, whereas on *The X Factor* they know they can sing and just get better. The other thing I watch is *Masterchef* because it makes me laugh. Like the time when John picked up a piece of black salmon and said, 'That's one well-cooked piece of fish.' What an understatement.

But maybe my favourite thing is a game called Boggle. It's a box full of letters that you jumble up to make words and I love it because it feels like there are lots of them inside me which I can see in the game. That's why I also enjoy reading because books are full of words you can lose yourself in. One I really like is Enid Blyton's *The Magic Faraway Tree*. It's for younger kids really but it's great because it tells the story of a group of friends who climb an enchanted tree and find a different land at the top of it each time. So they visit places like the Land of Spells, where they accidentally make a child shrink, the Land of Magic Medicines, where they buy a potion for their mum who's ill in bed, and the Land of Presents (that one's obvious).

The place I like the sound of best, though, is the Land of Do As You Please where the children get to do whatever they want –

like drive a train, ride elephants and swim in the sea. A lot of people think you stop having fun if you get sick, which means you never get to go to the Land of Do As You Please. But I know it's not like that. Sometimes you have to have fun in a different way, but mostly you have it just like other kids.

It's really important to have fun and I don't understand the adults who think their life is really bad. You've only got one and if you don't enjoy it then you've blown it, haven't you? That's why I always try to get to the Land of Do As You Please as often as possible (although it's much easier with the help of a Nintendo or *High School Musical* DVD or something).

You see, if I could have any wish it wouldn't be a year in Disneyland (although that would be nice) or a walk-on part in *High School Musical* (although that would be unreal). What I'd like is to live just one day without having to stop and rest when my heart gets tired: I'd go out and just waste my energy – visit Lucy's horses, ping all over the place doing stuff with friends, dance to *Mamma Mia*!

But I can't do that, and I've had to learn that feeling unhappy about it is a waste of time. Being happy gives me far more energy – so much so that sometimes I want to do a cartwheel even though I can't actually manage it. So that's how I try to feel each and every day, and I think I've always been like that. But I can't really remember that far back, so Mum will have to tell you more about how everything started.

❦ Kirsty ❦

I don't know how I knew it was the day on which our world would fall apart. Call it a mother's intuition, my medical training or just luck, but that day in December 1999 I knew I couldn't listen to another doctor telling me there was nothing wrong with Hannah.

'I want a second opinion,' I said to the young A&E doctor standing in front of me at Worcester Hospital.

Hannah was lying on a bed between us. She was pale and listless, so quiet. Not the bubbly, chatty four-year-old I knew so well. It was about 11 p.m. and she'd woken up a couple of hours before, crying and complaining of a tummy ache.

The doctor looked at me as exasperation washed across his face.

'You just need to give her some Calpol,' he said.

'I already have,' I lied.

I didn't want to be dismissed with paracetamol. I wasn't simply another over-protective mother. Someone had to listen to me. Something was terribly wrong. I knew it.

'I think you should take her home and see how she is in the morning,' the doctor replied slowly. 'You can always see the GP if she's still not feeling well tomorrow.'

I stared at the man, wanting to fly at him and scream.

'I want a second opinion,' I said in a low voice, trying to keep my rage under control.

'Well, I'm afraid there's no paediatric consultant on duty tonight. You'll have to take her to Birmingham or Hereford to be seen.'

'In an ambulance?'

'No.'

I didn't have time to argue. Scooping up Hannah in my arms, I ran out of A&E towards the car. Putting her into her seat, I ran around the car, got in and started the engine. Hereford was closer – 45 minutes' drive away.

'My tummy hurts, Mummy,' Hannah moaned.

'I know, darling, and we're going to make it better,' I said softly.

Hannah shut her eyes as I started driving. The minutes slid by as I turned over everything again and again. Why wouldn't the doctor listen to me? Why hadn't I done something more before now? Hannah hadn't been well for a few weeks but the GP had told me it was just a virus and I had listened as I told myself she was tired at the end of her first term at school. When she hadn't perked up, I'd gone back to the GP again and was told the same thing – she had one of those unspecific childhood bugs that every under-five gets and she'd soon shake it off.

So when Hannah had refused to eat on a visit to see my great aunt Kitty, I'd told her off. When bruises had appeared on the tops of her feet, I'd explained them away by a bang she'd got when she opened a cupboard door. I told myself I was being over-indulgent – the kind of mother who won't listen to good medical advice when she's given it. The kind of mother I didn't want to be. But what kind of mother was I now? I'd known deep down that something was wrong and hadn't trusted my own judgement. Now I knew I must.

Fear turned inside me as I drove and pressed my accelerator foot closer to the floor. Hedges and trees rushed by in the blackness as we neared Hereford.

'Nearly there, Han,' I said in the singsong voice mothers use to calm fear, anger or anything in between.

But Hannah did not reply and I turned to glance at her beside me. She looked as if she was sleeping. Reaching across, I grabbed her leg and shook it.

'Han?' I said. 'Han?'

She didn't open her eyes. I pushed my foot down harder, trying to stave off a rush of panic. Was she breathing? Should I stop to check? No. I didn't have time. I had to get her to hospital. They could do more for her there than I could.

Driving into the entrance of Hereford Hospital, I headed for the children's ward. I'd done some nursing shifts there before so I knew where it was. It was quicker than trying to find A&E. Hannah was limp in my arms as I pulled her out of the car. Quick, quick. Hurry. Let me in.

I hit the doorbell to the unit but nothing happened and I stared around me, ready to start screaming. But suddenly the door opened and I dashed inside. Running along the corridor, I could feel Hannah lying in my arms. My baby. My precious girl.

Flying towards the children's ward, I hit the bell on another door and waited for a voice to crackle out of the intercom. It seemed like for ever until it opened and I ran into a long corridor.

'I need help,' I pleaded as I reached the nursing station. 'Please. My daughter is unconscious.'

Nurses burst into life in front of me and Hannah was taken out of my arms. I followed as she was carried into a room. Very pale, her breathing was fast and shallow as a doctor started examining her. Please, please let her be OK. Make her well again.

'We'll need to put a line up,' the doctor said as the nurses peeled off the top of Hannah's cream all-in-one sleep suit.

I stared in horror at her tiny body. It was covered in tiny red marks – more appearing with each second – livid spots popping under her skin as if an invisible person was pricking her. The doctor pressed a needle into her right arm to take some blood.

'We'll send this straight off to the lab,' he said as he slipped the syringe into a plastic bag.

Hannah was still semi-conscious as she was put onto a saline drip. Now all we could do was wait for the blood test results. Time disappeared as I sat by her bed waiting. She looked so tiny – her blonde hair clinging to her head and her breathing still shallow and rapid. Her skin was so pale, it looked almost grey. I wanted to do something. Surely I could? I was her mother, the one person who would always protect her. But even as I tried telling myself this was some everyday, run-of-the-mill illness, I felt the spark of fear which lies inside every mother from the day their first child is born uncurl itself inside me.

'Mrs Jones?' a voice said. 'The doctor wants to speak to you.'

I was taken into a room where the doctor was waiting with a nurse. She walked towards me as if to put her arm around my shoulders but stopped as I stared at her. I knew what this meant. I'd seen it a lot during twelve years of nursing. But I'd always been on the other side before – one of the people waiting to gently break bad news to a stunned relative.

I sat down opposite the doctor.

'We've had the results back,' he said. 'I'm afraid Hannah is very poorly. Do you have any idea what is wrong with her?'

I looked at him. I'd been going over it in my mind and knew – the bruising, tiredness, loss of appetite. I should have realised before now.

'I think so,' I replied.

The doctor looked at me.

'Hannah has tummy ache because she's bleeding into her stomach and is now beginning to bleed everywhere. We need to work quickly to save her life now.'

I stayed silent as I listened.

'This is very serious, Mrs Jones,' the doctor continued softly. 'Hannah is a very sick little girl. We think she has leukaemia.'

It was quiet on the ward, past midnight, as I opened my eyes and looked at Hannah. A small light above her bed threw soft beams and shadows across it. Standing up, I tucked her yellow knitted blanket around her. We'd brought it from home – something familiar in all that was so new.

Turning around, I stared at the plastic chair which I'd earlier folded out flat before wrapping a hospital sheet and blanket around it. This was my bed now, but I knew I wouldn't be able to switch off as I lay down and heard the hushed sounds of the hospital at night – the clip of nurses' footsteps, the rumble of trolley wheels and the soft beeps made by machines. I felt as I had in the first few weeks after becoming a mother – too scared to fall properly asleep as I listened to Hannah breathing. Like all new mothers, mine had been a waking sleep all those years ago until I'd learned to trust the fact that she was safe. Now such certainty was gone.

Hours after arriving at Hereford, we'd been transferred to Birmingham Children's Hospital and already the map of our world was unrecognisable. Gone were pre-school and nursery pick-ups, bath times and stories before bed. Instead there were lumbar punctures and central lines, HB levels and platelets.

We'd been plunged into our new world during our first meeting with Hannah's oncology consultant, Dr Williams. Young, smiling and comfortably rounded, he'd told us that she had probable acute myeloid leukaemia – an aggressive and rarer form of the blood cancer. From that moment on there was a flurry of activity, questions and tests. This morning Hannah had gone down to the operating rooms to be anaesthetised for a lumbar puncture to confirm the diagnosis and identify the specific type of leukaemia by drawing spinal fluid to test for cancer cells. A central line had also been inserted – an intravenous catheter which snaked through her chest wall and into her jugular vein ready to deliver chemotherapy drugs straight to her heart.

Andrew and I had sat quietly as Mr Williams explained AML to us. In healthy adults and children, bone marrow produces red blood cells to carry oxygen around the body, white blood cells to fight infection and platelets to knit blood together and control bleeding. But in Hannah this system had gone out of control, like a rollercoaster crashing off its tracks into the unknown. Deep within the core of her bones, her marrow was over-producing imperfect cells. It meant that healthy blood was not being made which was why Hannah had started bleeding internally. Without treatment she would certainly die. With it, she stood a chance.

For a moment fear had engulfed me as the doctor talked – a bitter, clenching terror that filled my gut. But I'd pushed it down as I listened to every word he said, knowing I must keep myself calm as we prepared to fight for Hannah's life. Working for many years at the extreme end of nursing – intensive care and cardiac transplant wards, major injuries units and paediatric ICU transfer – had taught me how to do this. In the rush and panic of acute medicine I'd learned to keep still in the eye of a storm. Sick and infirm, young and fit, death was a random enemy which didn't make allowances as it took lives. But it was only now as it tried to take my own child that I knew what fear really tasted like.

It had all felt unreal during those first anxious hours in Hereford Hospital as we waited to be transferred to Birmingham by blue-light ambulance. After the doctor had spoken to me, I'd phoned Andrew and he'd arrived desperate for news, tears wet on his cheeks as both of us tried to take in what was happening. Until then we'd had an ordinary life: Andrew working as an auditor and me doing twenty hours a week as a junior sister on a coronary care unit in Worcester, juggling my shifts around our three children, babysitters and nursery. We lived in a new house on a little estate and went on holiday once a year. It was a busy, run-of-the-mill life until we stepped out of the lift into the long corridor leading through Birmingham's paediatric oncology unit for the first time and I knew nothing would ever be the same again.

Hannah was lying on a stretcher and I looked up to see a little girl walking towards us. She must have been about ten and was stick thin – a pair of shorts hanging from her hips and a white T-shirt dropping in folds around her body, her head completely bald. She looked like a ghost as she pushed a drip stand, and my breath caught as I stared at her. Just the day before I'd been planning for Christmas because it was only a week away. What toys to buy? What food to cook? Did I have enough to fill the children's stockings? Did I have too much? But now this world had disappeared completely and it had taken just one word to shatter it. Four syllables. Leu-kae-mi-a.

As Mr Williams talked us through Hannah's diagnosis and treatment, he'd shown us a red file containing pages of tiny typed words listing all the different forms of chemotherapy and their side effects. Hannah's leukaemia would be treated by six rounds of chemo which would last about a month each and all follow the same pattern – after an initial burst of intensive drugs over several days, Hannah would continue on a lighter cocktail of medication for another ten before being given a 'rest' of about another ten days to allow her body to recover from the onslaught. It was like a war: a period of intense battle followed by a retreat and regrouping before the fighting began again. All we could do was wait to see if it would be enough to save Hannah's life.

'We hope Hannah will quickly go into remission,' Mr Williams had told us. 'But even if she does she will have to complete all six chemo courses to give her the best possible chance of long-term remission.'

Andrew and I had listened as Mr Williams warned us of the possible side effects the powerful chemo drugs could trigger because they would attack the healthy fast-growing cells in Hannah's skin and digestive tract as well as the cancerous ones. The chemo might cause anything from hair loss and nausea to skin changes and tiredness. Hannah's immune system would be so depleted by the highly toxic drugs that any tiny infection could be serious.

There was also the possibility of more extreme side effects like an increased risk of thrombosis or heart damage. But they were remote – the stuff of warnings listed on an aeroplane safety card which you barely glance at as you settle back in your seat. We didn't have a choice. We had to fight the enemy that was here and now. If Hannah didn't have the drugs, we would certainly lose her.

'I don't feel well, Mummy,' she'd cried when she'd woken up after Andrew and I had returned to her bedside. 'My tummy hurts.'

She'd hardly been awake since the night before. Too ill and drowsy to know what was happening.

'We're in hospital, darling,' I said softly as I bent towards her. 'You're poorly.'

She stared at me.

'There are bugs in your blood and the doctors are going to give you special medicines to fight them.'

Hannah looked at Andrew and me, her eyes huge in her white face.

'Will they taste nice?' she asked.

'These are special medicines which you don't have to swallow,' I replied.

'Will they make me better?'

I paused for a moment. I had a choice now: lace the truth with uncertain hopes or speak it gently but honestly on this, my first step into the unknown with my daughter. Hannah had to trust me completely. I couldn't start lying to her now.

'We don't know for sure, but we hope so, Han.'

Andrew and I looked at each other. There was nothing more to say.

~

As soon as Hannah started chemotherapy, it quickly became clear just how much the treatment was going to affect her. The chemotherapy drugs had to be administered day and night through two bags labelled with words like 'Toxic' which hung from drip stands beside her. Each ran in turn down the central line into Hannah's heart, which was washed out with saline whenever the drugs were switched to ensure they did not mix. Within days, she had started passing blood clots or vomiting them up as the skin on her inner digestive tract disintegrated.

It is one thing knowing your child must have life-saving treatment but another to watch them have it. The cries of children too young to understand what was happening cut razor-sharp through me and at nights the buzz of the day disappeared and soft sobs filled the silence. But the only time Hannah cried out was when the drips and lines going into her veins caught as they were moved. Otherwise she lay still and her silence was almost worse than screams. It was as if she was too sick to even make a sound, too weak to express her pain in any way, and I wished I could climb inside her mind and know what she was thinking.

Time disappeared. I didn't think of the next chemo cycle, next month or even next week. I knew Oli and Lucy were being looked after at home by Andrew and his parents so I focused completely on Hannah. My days were lived waiting for her latest blood results: white and red blood cell counts, platelet levels and HB ratings. Leucocytes, basophils, eosinophils, creatinine levels … the list of blood cells and other physiological markers was endless. Each morning a blood sample was taken, and after the results came back soon after lunch I'd write down the figures in a pocket-sized book – lines of numbers running like Chinese shupai down the page which told me about the minutest details of my child's fight with the disease inside her.

The tiny figures became my talismen and I'd wait anxiously each day until the small hand hit the number two on my watch face and it was time to walk to the nurses' station to ask for news.

'It must be busy in the labs today,' someone would smile. 'They'll be here soon.'

Pushing down my impatience, I'd walk back to Hannah's bed. But in my desperation for news I wasn't any different from every other mum on the ward who also pored over the figures when they got them. Did their child have an infection? Was their red blood count coming back up? Or their white count going down? Some couldn't decipher the list of intricate numbers and asked me to explain after realising

I could help. I understood why they wanted to know what the endless figures meant: they were the one piece of fact we could hold onto amid so much uncertainty, and understanding the numbers felt like some small practical way to help our child at a time when there was so little else we could do.

Otherwise I spent hours sitting beside Hannah, longing to get onto her bed and lie beside her like other parents did with their children but unable to because she didn't want to be touched. Hannah's senses were so heightened that her skin was incredibly sensitive and I found it hard not to physically reassure her. I wanted to cradle her just as I had when she was a baby, feel her weight against me and soothe her. But Hannah did not want to be hugged and she did not cry out for me either. She lay in a cocoon of silence, as if willing herself to live, while I sat within arm's reach, close enough for her to feel my presence. The hours slipped by with the television on low as she slept and when she woke I would colour in a picture so that she could watch, or read a story for her to listen to.

Too ill to eat, Hannah was fed by a high-calorie feed which dripped slowly into her nasogastric tube from another bag on a drip stand beside the bed. Thick and sticky, the feed had to be covered in brown paper to protect it from the sun because light could alter its delicate chemical balance and we quickly got used to this strange kind of nourishment, just as we did the rest of our new life. After that first shocking sight of the little girl walking towards me, it soon became normal to see children with no hair; after a few nights in the chair beside

Hannah's bed I knew other parents in the ward were lying awake just like me and occasionally I could hear their muffled sobs. We smiled at each other during the day and silently accepted each other's grief by night.

~

Life on the unit wasn't just about sadness – there was hope and light too. Doctors walked around in white coats splattered with water shot from pistols by the children who were well enough to play, and the nurses, who worked harder than any I'd ever seen, were endlessly cheerful. Christmas also worked its magic on the ward just as surely as it did in any other place filled with children. Decorations were strung across the walls, nurses played carols on the radio and Father Christmas visited the children each day to hand out presents. If Hannah was sleeping when he came, she'd wake to see a Barbie car or a colouring book, a doll or a fairy wand, in the stack of presents which slowly piled up beside her bed.

I liked the fact that the doctors who clustered around her each morning to assess her progress – the consultant Dr Williams, a registrar, senior and junior house officers and various medical students – were followed by a man with a red jacket and a huge smile. Just like every other four-year-old, Hannah loved Father Christmas, and although she was too sick to express her excitement I knew she enjoyed his visits each day.

He was something comfortingly familiar – just like the duvet, sheets and pillows Andrew had brought from home after Hannah had told me the hospital ones were too scratchy. To minimise the risk of infection on a ward full of children who were so weak, I had to wash the linen each day to stop bugs breeding and soon realised we needed more supplies to keep up with the constant flow of clean laundry. But I knew the familiar smell of our washing powder would comfort Hannah, just as Father Christmas would – a bright spot in the day, a few moments for her to forget.

But after nearly a week in hospital a nurse came to deliver bad news just as Andrew arrived with Oli and Lucy.

'There won't be a visit from you-know-who this afternoon,' she said in a low voice. 'There's no one to do it, unfortunately.'

I looked at Andrew – with his big belly and smiling eyes he'd be perfect for the job.

'Will the costume fit me?' he asked as he looked at the nurse.

'Size nine boots OK?'

'I'll squeeze into them.'

The nurse took Andrew off to get dressed as I turned to Oli and Lucy and breathed in their comforting smell while I cuddled them – Oli, a toddler of nearly three, and Lucy, a bouncing baby of fifteen months. I had missed them so much, and seeing the energy and life shining out of them was like seeing shards of light glittering across water – something everyday suddenly become magical.

'Where's Daddy?' Oli asked as he looked up from the colouring book he'd found.

'He's gone to the car to get something. He won't be long. Shall we draw a picture for him?'

Oli picked up some crayons as I jiggled Lucy, happy to feel her in my arms again, and waited for Andrew to come onto the ward. But as I watched him walk up to the first bed I suddenly realised that I might have made a mistake. Would Hannah recognise her father? She was an intelligent child, advanced beyond her years in many ways after being diagnosed with dyspraxia when she was two and a half. The condition was a bit like dyslexia but affected movement and coordination. It meant that Hannah had been late learning to walk and dress herself, but her language, as if in compensation, had developed quickly and she was also very sensitive to other people's emotions. Hannah could say 'octopus' before her first birthday and have long conversations about the plants in the garden by the time she was four. When my granny had fallen over one day while they were out for a walk she'd even calmly insisted to a passer-by that she could look after her.

But it was too late to do anything now because Andrew was walking up to Hannah's bed and all I could do was hope that she didn't recognise him as he chuckled, 'Ho, ho, ho'.

'Father Christmas!' Oli squealed as he jumped up.

I got up with Lucy as Andrew sat down on the chair beside Hannah's bed and Oli climbed onto his knee, listing the presents he wanted while Lucy sat in my arms, refusing to go anywhere near the strange man in red. When Andrew had finished with Oli, he turned to Hannah and held out his left hand towards her. She looked at him silently and I held my breath.

Very slowly, she lifted her right arm and pushed her hand into the space between the bed and chair where her father's was waiting for hers. Their fingers met in mid-air.

'You're being a very good little girl,' Andrew said softly.

Hannah's mouth curved into a tiny smile as she looked at Father Christmas and I knew this one piece of magic was still safe for her.

～

It was New Year's Eve 1999 – millennium night – and after two weeks in hospital the intensive phase of Hannah's first cycle of chemotherapy drugs had ended a few days before. But while I could hear people getting ready to celebrate outside on the streets of Birmingham, inside the hospital everything was quiet as Hannah lay almost unconscious. Two mornings ago the nurses had noticed her vital statistics weren't normal when they did her usual observations – her pulse was rising, her blood pressure and oxygen saturation were dropping. The doctors knew immediately that Hannah's heart was struggling and a cardiologist who'd seen her had told me she might be suffering a temporary side effect of the chemo. She'd been put on new medication but Hannah was still dangerously ill and was now on morphine to control her pain.

As the soft thud of music from outside weaved through our hushed world, I thought of all the people getting ready to see in midnight and wished Hannah could be among them, ruddy faced and smiling. Then I thought of Andrew and the children at home and sadness filled me that we wouldn't be celebrating this milestone together as a family. Instead we were far apart and Hannah was lying still on the bed with her eyes closed, barely conscious, oblivious to the nasal canula running underneath her nose to give her oxygen, the feeding tube running up it or the central line attached to her chest. Three sticky electrode pads were attached to a heart monitor which beeped softly and a SATS probe on her finger constantly checked her oxygen levels.

All I could do was pray as I sat beside her, willing her back to consciousness. I felt angry and disappointed. How could this be happening to Hannah when she already had so much else to fight? After the hustle and bustle, the rush of emergency when we had first arrived in hospital, the silence now felt overwhelming and all the questions I had been asked since that day rolled in a constant stream through my mind.

There had been so many of them. Did I breastfeed? What type of bottled milk did I use? Did I warm it in the microwave? None are proven links to leukaemia, but as I searched for a reason why Hannah was now even sicker I focused on the questions I'd been asked and why. Surely I should have been able to stop the unseen enemy which had sneaked into our life? I must have made some mistake and allowed it in. Hannah was my child. My job was to protect her.

The questions almost consumed me – my mind going back and forth as I looked back on our life and tried to pinpoint where I'd gone wrong. I remembered how I'd only breastfed Hannah for a couple of weeks after she was born because I'd gone back to work. I hadn't had a choice about it, but now I wondered if I'd harmed her in some unthinking way at the very beginning of her life.

I'd longed to be a mother when I'd met Andrew eight years before. I was twenty-five and knew I was ready to fall in love and start my own family after returning from a year travelling in Australia. I'd been brought up by my grandmother after my mother had died when I was five, and although my childhood had been strict but loving, the loss had implanted in me a need to create the bustling family life I hadn't had. My childhood was one of such stillness and routine that I craved a big, messy family full of life and laughter.

I'd met Andrew in a village pub where he'd stood out a mile in his suit. Quiet and kind, he was a big man who made me feel safe and when I got home after our first date, I told my grandmother I was going to marry him – even if he didn't know it yet. I proposed four months later but Andrew refused because it was too soon and I was being typically impetuous. So we waited another year to get engaged and I was over the moon when we started trying for a baby.

But two years had passed and I hadn't fallen pregnant. No one could explain why, and I felt hopelessness seep into me for the first time in my life as the months turned into years. Feeling more and more overwhelmed, I gave up my job and stayed in bed for weeks until realising I couldn't lie there forever. So I forced myself back out into the world, where I got a job on a production line at a cake factory – repetitive, undemanding work that I didn't need to worry about – and told myself I would fall pregnant when the time was right. Two months later I did, and was overjoyed. My family was finally starting and I knew I'd do anything to protect it.

So when Andrew had been made redundant weeks before Hannah was born I had found a job to support us and returned to work when she was just three and a half weeks old. But leaving her was even worse than I had anticipated because I was soon sent to a conference in Canada by the pharmaceutical company I was working for. I ached every day for Hannah, who was being looked after by Andrew and my grandmother, and was overjoyed when he found a new job. It meant I could go home again and I'd stayed there ever since – first with Hannah, then Oli and Lucy – concentrating on our family life and working part-time as a nurse to help pay the bills.

But now, as I thought back to those few weeks of her life and tried to make sense of what was happening, I wondered if leaving Hannah was just the first mistake I'd made without even knowing it.

The world closed down to just Hannah and me – she and I in a silent bubble together as we fought her illness, travelling a path that seemed to get darker and darker. Three days into the New Year she was transferred into the high dependency unit – a halfway house between the oncology wards and intensive care.

Semi-conscious and still on morphine, we lived in half-darkness, blinds closed and wave sounds playing softly to soothe Hannah. Various different types of therapy were offered to children by aromatherapists and reflexologists who came onto the ward. But all they could do for Hannah was give her crystals – pebble-smooth stones that we put in the palms of her hands as she lay in bed hardly moving.

We were closer to the edge of darkness than ever before, and for the first time the word 'die' whispered around the edges of my thoughts. Before now I'd refused to let myself think it, pushed it out as I concentrated on Hannah's treatment. But now I knew I couldn't ignore it any longer as she lay silently. No one knew for sure yet why Hannah had so suddenly weakened and, desperate to try and make some sense of the chaos inside me, I had asked for a priest to come and perform the Anointing of the Sick – prayers said for those who are dangerously ill. I had been brought up with a strong Catholic faith and Hannah had always enjoyed church. She'd also liked the nuns who visited the children's ward so much that she'd ask where they were if we hadn't seen them for a few days. Hannah liked routine and they always came on time before reading the same prayers, exuding a quiet stillness which calmed her.

Now I watched the priest as he softly traced the sign of the cross on Hannah's forehead.

'Through this holy anointing, may the Lord in his love and mercy help you with the grace of the Holy Spirit,' he said softly.

Hannah did not move or speak but her eyes were open as she watched. The familiar words and phrases of the prayers felt soothing – just as knowing other people were praying for us was. When Hannah had first been admitted to hospital, my great aunt Kitty, who had once been a nun, had contacted all the churches she knew and by now hundreds of people were praying for Hannah. It comforted me to know that we were not alone.

After the priest gave me communion and left, I sat down again, lost in thought as Hannah slept. Ever since becoming an adult, I'd been making plans and being busy – first with my career, then meeting Andrew, next came buying a home and finally starting our family. Now I had three children under five to keep me constantly busy and I hurled myself through the hours each day, waiting for the next child's cry when they fell over or a frustrated howl as they couldn't complete a task.

But now for the first time ever there was no shift to start at work, cleaning to do, food shopping to get or another child to calm. All I could do was concentrate on tiny things: the feel of Hannah's right hand enclosed in my left one as it lay limply on the bed. It felt so small, as fragile as a shell hurled across a windswept beach, and I focused on the feel of it in mine – the one fixed point in a landscape which seemed to change almost by the hour.

It isn't just emotional certainties you lose when your child falls sick and your world spins off its axis, it is practical ones too – the thousand tiny tasks which make up the physically demanding job of being a mother. Of course you willingly hand over their care to the doctors and nurses trying to save their life. But in doing so, the daily throwaway acts which have made up your life ever since your child came into it are suddenly no longer yours and you realise, for perhaps the first time, that these are the things which make you a mother – loading a dishwasher, wiping a face or turning book pages, each one giving you a purpose and reason which you feel lost without.

I clung to the little things I could still do – checking Hannah's feeding tubes, smoothing her sheets or wiping her hands clean of the blood spots running off the drips – but knew it wasn't practical care she needed from me any more.

Hannah and I had moved beyond an everyday world of yoghurt pots and finger painting, cut knees and spilt drinks. We'd fallen off the map into the lands where dragons lay.

But as I sat with her, I realised that I must conquer my fears if I was to be what I hoped for Hannah. I had to stop looking back at the past and searching for a reason where there was none. She needed my courage, reassurance and strength to draw on more than ever now – a fixed point in all the uncertainty. I could not dwell on making sense of the past or controlling the uncertain future. I must live in the moment, finding strength in it and living it with Hannah, knowing it was precious minute by minute, hour by hour and day by day.

I had always been so busy focusing on goals and the next plan. Upgrading cars, booking holidays, finding schools – like many people I'd been preoccupied with a future that was just beyond my reach, hardly taking any notice of the moment I was in. But as Hannah's life hung in the balance I finally saw what I could lose if I wasted the moment. Each one was precious and I wanted her to feel loved in them all.

Hannah herself was helping me to see this. Ever since she'd fallen ill she had quietly accepted what was happening, and her calmness had humbled me. She hadn't questioned the drugs or railed against the endless tests. She hadn't complained when she was in pain or screamed at the injustice of it all. She had simply submitted herself to what was happening and in doing so had guided me as much as I had guided her as we took uncertain steps through our new world. I knew that Hannah might die and had to accept the possibility, however much I didn't want to. But the strength she needed from me would not come from looking back or forward. I must live in the moment with her – cling to each one and treasure it. As I sat with Hannah, I knew this was a lesson she was helping me to learn. But what I did not know then was that it would be just the first of many.

CHAPTER TWO

Precious Time

❀

It was Dad's birthday a few days ago and we went out for a meal at a pub to celebrate last night. Mum and Dad, Oli, Lucy, Phoebe and me went as well as Grandma and Granddad, my Uncle Nigel, Auntie Serena and my cousins Katie, who is ten, and Toby, who's a bit younger than Phoebe. Becky, our friend who used to live over the road from us, also came with her mum Lindy and sister Abby. We all gave Dad his presents when we got to the pub and I'd made him a card using a craft kit which I'd covered in hearts and flowers. I also got him a tie and some chocolates because he loves those.

I got to dress up especially to go out because earlier this week I went into town with £40 that I'd saved up from my pocket money. I don't often look around the shops but I was really looking forward to going and seeing what there was. I'm awful at making up my mind, though, so I went from shop to shop before going back to the first place to buy the first thing I saw. I always do that because I have to be sure that what I think I like is what I really want. So when I was finally certain, I bought some gold sandals I'd seen in the first shop. It's still only April and my feet might get a bit cold when I wear them but they're really nice. I'd like to have heels but can only wear flat shoes because my balance isn't good enough for high ones. Lucy has got some platforms but they make me fall over.

Lucy and I were so excited about going out for Dad's birthday that we started getting ready yesterday afternoon. We've both got makeup and so I did hers before painting her nails. Then she did my toes but I did my fingers because she makes them too messy. Mum doesn't usually like us wearing makeup but we're allowed to on special occasions. The trouble was that we were ready by 3 p.m. and so Mum sent me to bed to have a rest. She said I'd be too tired if I didn't sleep and I knew she was right, but it was still boring.

I got out of bed just before we left and had roast chicken, chips, peas and a knickerbocker glory at the pub. Then we sang 'Happy Birthday' to Dad as a waitress brought his pudding with a candle in it. That was when the fun really started because some of our friends were on a big table behind us. They're called Tina and Marco and they own an equestrian centre near our house where Lucy and Mum go riding sometimes.

Everything was normal until suddenly a rolled-up napkin landed on the table in front of Lucy and me. We looked around and Marco was laughing, so we lobbed one back. That was it. Marco threw another napkin, Mum chucked one back at him and then Marco flicked a pea which flew over my head and landed on the table. Lucy and I were really laughing by now as I threw a piece of bread. Then suddenly Tina, her daughter Emma and another little girl I didn't know all joined in. Everyone was at it until Dad got cross and told Lucy and me to stop.

'You should know better, Hannah,' Dad said, and I knew he was angry because the people who own the pub are his friends.

Mum started clearing up bits of napkin and bread while Dad stomped off back to the car. But instead of feeling bad, I felt annoyed because I was the one getting all the blame even though it wasn't all my fault. That always happens. Lucy and I can be nutty when we're together, and once when Dad sent us to our bedrooms we hid in hers and decided that we were going to put Mum's knickers on our head, bang all the saucepans together and do karaoke so loud that Dad couldn't hear the TV. We didn't do any of it in the end but I'm sure I'd have got the blame if we had because I'm the oldest. It really annoys me.

So I was feeling angry until I got in the car, and Dad was quiet. Then I started feeling bad because I realised that I'd ruined his party. I felt worse and worse until we got home and I went to bed which was where Mum found me crying when she came in to say goodnight.

'I've messed everything up,' I told her. 'And I've been told off twice. I know when I've ruined things.'

(I'd actually only been told off once by Dad, but I thought Mum was going to as well when she came in to see me so I added that in.) But then Mum told me not to worry and that Dad was fine – everything had been cleared up and no harm had been done – which is when I got angry again. I knew Mum was trying to make me feel not too bad, which was nice of her, but everyone has to feel sorry sometimes and so do I. It annoys me when people treat me differently and that's why I didn't like Mum doing it because one of the best things about my family is that I'm normal to them which makes up for all the people who give me the Chitty Chitty Bang Bang look. Remember how scared the baroness was when the children took over her castle? How she screamed at the sight of them? Well, that's how some people look at me and it's the worst – worse even than when Dad gets a face like thunder if we interrupt his rugby game on TV – and the reason I hate it is because I know the person giving it to me doesn't see me as a normal teenager.

Now I know I'm not exactly average: I'm thirteen and I've been in and out of hospital all my life. But the Chitty Chitty Bang Bang look tells me I'm abnormal, and while I know I'm a bit different I'm not a total weirdo. That's why I like my mates so much because they never look at me like that, and that's why I got so angry when Mum tried to make me feel better because it made me feel like it does when a teacher gives out homework at school before saying to me: 'Do as much as you can.' They usually say it quietly but even if everyone has left the class I reckon people are still in the corridor so they can hear. When a teacher says that I'm like, 'Whatever! I can't run a race but I can do my schoolwork.' (Actually, I don't say that but I shout it in my head.)

It's not that I want to do homework or anything. In fact, I hated homework from the moment I started going to school when I was nearly ten. I had not been to school since I was sick as a little girl, and me and homework didn't get on because when

I got home it was dinner time, TV and bed. There was no time for homework and I don't understand why kids have to do it anyway because we're at school for more than half the day which should be enough. But even though I hate it, I hate it more when a teacher makes out that I don't have to do it because I don't want to be treated any differently to anyone else.

So I was still angry when Mum left my bedroom and Dad came in to say goodnight. But then he told me he'd had a nice time and I promised I wouldn't throw napkins again when we went out, so I felt better. And I know it's good that Mum and Dad tell me off even though it's bad, if you see what I mean. It shows that they're not going to tiptoe around me like some people do. It's always been that way, and although I can't remember much about being in hospital with leukaemia Mum has told me that she even got cross with me back then because I kicked a doctor. I couldn't believe I'd done that! But she's right to get angry sometimes because if people were nice to me all the time I'd have them wrapped around my little finger. I'd be able to do exactly what I want and there have to be rules otherwise I wouldn't get anywhere. Things would also fall apart in our house because there are four kids here.

It's a bit like *Wind in the Willows* when Badger tries to get Toad out of his obsession with cars. Toad is doing all sorts of stupid things and Badger tells him it's got to stop. But Toad doesn't listen so they lock him up in his room and he climbs out of the window, escapes and ends up in prison. It's not until near the end of the book that he realises Badger was right and he was wrong.

The problem is that Toad doesn't have any discipline, and look where he ends up. He has to learn that there are different kinds of discipline too: the bigger one that stops you from chucking napkins around because other people will get angry and the smaller one that stops you from doing things which aren't good for you. I had to learn that one when I first came out of hospital after saying no to a heart transplant because while I was in bed most of the time at first, my energy got bigger and bigger as I got stronger. But then I realised that if I did too much I'd feel ill again, so I had to learn not to even though I wanted to go mad. I had to save my energy so I could do stuff later like wind Phoebe up otherwise my blood pressure would drop and I'd see funny lights in front of my eyes.

It was really hard because sometimes I wanted to get up so much that I almost had to ask Mum to pin me down. But eventually I taught myself to stay still even though being bored and tired is the worst thing in the world for me. Being bored and tired is worse than salmon, swordfish, prawns in mayonnaise, my computer crashing or even getting cold when I go outside and knowing I have to go back in again because I've had it.

Being bored and tired is worse than all of those, but I've had to learn that I must lie down until the tiredness goes away because that's the only way I'm going to feel better, even if it takes days. That's why discipline is important, that's what Toad didn't learn until it was almost too late and that's why I'm glad Dad told me off last night.

If he didn't do it sometimes then I'd run rings around him and Mum like I've seen some children do in hospital. I knew one girl who refused to eat anything except crisps and I realised that it's easy to get spoiled if you're sick and I'm glad I haven't been. My mum and dad have made me happy but I don't think I'm a spoiled child. Getting told off occasionally makes me feel normal, and I like that. It's really important.

‘I don't want any more medicine,’ Hannah whispered as I bent towards her.

‘You must, Han. It will make you better.’

‘I don't want it,’ she said with a sob. ‘I'm tired.’

‘I know, Han, but soon you'll have had enough medicines and then you'll be able to play again.’

Hannah's eyes were uncertain as she looked at me.

‘Would you like me to read you a story?’ I asked softly.

‘No.’

‘Are you sure?’

‘Yes. I'm busy.’

‘Doing what, Han?’

‘Fighting all the bugs.’

Hannah had regained consciousness soon after New Year, and days later we'd learned that she had gone into remission. It was wonderful news because it meant there were no cancer cells in her blood. But remission isn't a cure and in a way there's no such thing when it comes to the unpredictable foe that is cancer. Like every other patient, it was simply a question of time for Hannah – five years of remission was the benchmark of true hope, five years before we could believe with any certainty that she was really well – and even though her remission was a good start, we could not draw quiet confidence from it because the problems with Hannah's heart had still not been solved. In fact, they had worsened during the second chemo cycle and were only just being controlled by medication as the doctors tried to decide what was happening.

They knew for sure that a virus wasn't causing the problem and had adjusted Hannah's medications to keep her stable. But she had developed septicaemia which was putting extra pressure on her heart and still needed to complete all six chemo cycles to maximise her chances of being well in the long term. Andrew and I had been shown charts mapping the recurrence rates of leukaemia and seen for ourselves in black and white the lines on the graphs which dived down dramatically the more chemo a patient had.

I knew Andrew found the situation very hard. He struggled with the fact that we were not being given definite answers about Hannah's heart, but I understood that medicine was often more of an art than a science, a piecing together of clues before coming to a conclusion based on instinct instead of certainty. It takes time to make a diagnosis in such a complex situation, and I trusted the doctors to do all they could to find out what was wrong.

In the meantime, we'd stayed in the high dependency unit for Hannah's second round of chemo to allow the doctors to keep a close eye on her, and this time the drugs had taken an even greater toll on her body than before. As they worked their way into her system, Hannah started being sick up to six times a day and had terrible diarrhoea. Her fingernails and toenails had also fallen out to reveal raw red nail beds which I dressed each day with tiny pieces of paraffin gauze which had been chilled in the fridge. Wrapping them loosely around her finger and toe tips, I would bandage each one as she cried out softly. She also needed gauze pads placed under her heels, shoulder blades and bottom to stop sores developing because her skin was peeling – the new skin so painful that she had to be handled like a burns victim. For several days we could hardly touch Hannah because she was in too much pain, and even her mouth bled – blood caking her gums, teeth and lips which I tried to wipe gently away.

As I did so, I wondered how high a price anyone could pay for being cured, let alone a child. Hannah was wracked with pain, and although I wished I could feel it for her, I couldn't. Doubts and distress filled me as I watched her suffer. Sick and exhausted, she lay in bed as the drugs worked their way through her body – her face the chalk white of marble, the only movement coming from pink tears which trickled from the corners of her eyes because her mucous membranes were so fragile that tiny spots of blood had seeped into them. Silently, Hannah would cry tears the colour of sunsets which left red crackled lines behind on her pale skin – the fragile markings of her pain.

I bled with Hannah too. Soon after Christmas I'd discovered I was pregnant with my fourth child and was pleased despite everything. I knew it was a bad time and people would wonder how we'd ever cope, but I felt that any life was a blessing and this one was no different. Soon after finding out, though, I had started bleeding and knew I was miscarrying. I told myself the baby had died for a reason and I needed all my strength to look after Hannah. But as I looked at her pink tears, I didn't know if I could believe in reason any more. What was happening to her simply didn't make sense.

Hannah sat in the middle of the towel-covered bed. The drugs for her second chemo cycle had finished last week and the curtains were drawn around her bed as a nurse stood in front of us holding a pair of hair clippers.

The previous day Hannah had looked into a tiny pink Barbie mirror before turning to face me.

'I look like Bert,' she'd said. 'Can I be like the others, please?'

Bert was one of her favourite *Sesame Street* characters, and I knew what Hannah meant. Many of the children on the oncology unit had completely lost their hair and she had obviously had enough of being only halfway through the process. I was glad she was telling me what she wanted again because it meant the little girl I knew was coming back to me.

'Of course we can give you a haircut, my darling,' I said. 'Shall we ask a nurse to do it?'

'Yes, please.'

I knew I couldn't bring myself to do it. Hannah's pale gold hair had always framed her beautiful blue eyes and I didn't feel able to rid her of it when only weeks before I'd tied it back into bunches and plaits ready for school. It had felt like such a milestone when she started, as if she was moving a step in front of me to venture out into the wide world – the beginning of the rest of her life.

'This won't take a minute,' the nurse said with a smile as she stepped towards the bed.

Hannah had seemed excited as we'd planned her hair 'cut' but now didn't look so sure as the clippers' harsh metallic buzz filled the room. She was silent as the nurse started cutting and I stood motionless as the last of Hannah's hair started to fall to the floor and tears ran down her face.

'I want my hair,' she said with a sob.

I longed to comfort her, to tell the nurse to stop even as I made myself smile brightly to try and calm her.

'Nearly there, Han,' I whispered. 'Soon you can try on one of your pretty hats.'

I'd bought a couple that I hoped she might like – a straw boater covered with flowers, a red chequered baseball cap and a pink beanie made of soft sweatshirt material.

Hannah was quiet again until the clippers finally fell silent and I looked at my child transformed. Her head was completely bald and her eyes looked even bigger in her gaunt face as she lifted her hand to touch her naked skull – an almost questioning gesture, like a toddler reaching out a tentative foot as they try to climb a step for the first time.

'Which hat would you like?' I asked.

Hannah pointed at the boater and I slipped it onto her head.

'It's too itchy,' she said.

'Silly Mummy,' I said as I took off the boater.

I hadn't thought of how straw would feel on newly bare skin. There were so many things to learn.

'Can I try on the pink one?' she asked.

'Of course you can.'

I slipped the beanie onto her head.

'That's better,' Hannah said, and smiled. 'My head's not cold any more.'

Oli's third birthday was in late January, and after almost six weeks in hospital with Hannah I was desperate to try and get home for it. I thought of him and Lucy all the time: as I woke in the morning and wondered if they were still sleeping; as I ate my lunch from a hospital tray and hoped Andrew had persuaded them to eat their vegetables; when I heard the sounds of a TV programme Oli liked and imagined him watching it; or when a baby brother or sister came onto the ward and I thought of Lucy's smiles.

We saw them every other weekend and they'd also come to stay with us for a night. But it wasn't a great success because Lucy had been in Hannah's bed and Oli was beside me on the pull-out so no one was comfortable. But I couldn't bring myself to use the family suite because it meant leaving Hannah on the ward overnight and we both felt anxious if we were apart too long, as if the million invisible strands joining us were strained by distance.

But I was nevertheless aware that children's lives move fast because things had already changed. I had been sitting by

Hannah's bed one day when I looked up to see Lucy toddling towards me. She'd been on the cusp of walking for a while but my heart missed a beat as I realised I had not been there for her first steps. It was a moment that could never be recaptured, which was why I wanted to be at home so much for Oli's birthday. Hannah was also going to make the journey with me because, although very weak, the doctors thought she could manage the short trip and I'd been on and off the phone all week organising Oli's party. He'd asked for a pirate theme and I'd arranged for a bouncy castle to be put up in the garden. I'd also managed to slip out of the hospital for a couple of hours to buy pirate hats and party bags. Now Hannah seemed as excited as I was that we were going home.

'What presents will Oli have?' she kept asking as we waited for Andrew to pick us up.

'Pirate ones!' I exclaimed with a smile.

We were all a little quiet on the ninety-minute journey home and after pulling onto the drive, Andrew lifted Hannah out of the car to take her inside. I followed behind and stepped over the threshold to smell a different home. Everything was spotless – even the black-and-white checked kitchen floor that was usually covered in paint splashes and crumbs. I knew Andrew and his parents had gone to a lot of trouble, but I felt strange – like an animal that's gone back to its lair to find the scent of a stranger there. My home felt different now that I was not in it.

'Mummeeeeeee,' Oli shouted as he ran towards me. 'Look at the food. Have you got my present? When does the party start?'

I felt a rush of pleasure to see him so excited as he took my hand to lead me into the garden and look at the bouncy castle. But as we walked outside I suddenly felt anxious. Was Hannah OK? I took a deep breath as I told myself she would be fine. Andrew was looking after her now. This was my time with Oli. He deserved that.

As the party got under way the house filled with children and parents and I went to get Hannah from the lounge to carry her into the kitchen. I wanted her to feel part of the day, not separated from it, and I sat her on the work surface so she could look out of the window at the children playing in the back garden – a gaggle of three-year-olds oblivious to the chill as they flung themselves on and off the bouncy castle. Their cheeks were pink and their laughter echoed through the frozen air as their mothers chatted to each other.

Hannah sat on the kitchen worktop beside me and I looked at her sitting quietly. Tiny veins covered her bald head, a transparent feeding tube snaked across her pale cheek up her nose, an oxygen tube ran under it and two drip stands stood like sentinels at a gate beside her. There were moments when she looked almost old and wizened, as if the weight of the treatment was too much for her to bear. Soon she would need another dose of heart medication.

'It's too cold for me in the garden, isn't it, Mummy?' Hannah said as she stared outside.

I looked at her, not sure what to say. I knew how much she wanted to play, to be a little girl again.

'Yes, my darling,' I said softly. 'But you can stay in here with me and I'll watch with you.'

Hannah sat still and quiet as she gazed at her brother playing with his friends. But just before we set off back to the hospital, Andrew cleared the bouncy castle and I carried her outside. It was freezing cold as I stepped gingerly across the garden with Hannah in my arms. She felt so fragile, like a baby wrapped up against the elements. Lifting her gently, I sat her on the edge of the bouncy castle and kneeled down to look at her. She didn't have the strength to make herself bounce and I knew she wouldn't want to. But Hannah was smiling as she sat quietly – staring at the grass, feeling the wind on her face and breathing in the world.

&

It wasn't just the doctors and nurses on the oncology ward who were filled with energy, kindness and patience. Many others worked with them to make life on the ward more bearable and perhaps the most inventive were the play leaders who found something to make even the sickest children smile. If a boy or girl was lying in bed and crying, a play leader would slide wax paper under their cheeks to catch their tears and show them the pattern they had made on the paper – a spidery trail of drops and wiggling lines to make them smile – or if a child was too weak to move, they would make a shape out of play dough and put it into their hand so their fingers could curl around it. They seemed to possess a never-ending treasure chest of ideas to help children smile and Hannah always looked forward to their visits.

There was one in particular though who could always make her laugh and Hannah's favourite game with Sarah involved dipping sponges into water before lying in wait for a doctor to pass the bed.

'Go on!' Sarah would shriek and Hannah would toss the wet sponge at the unsuspecting passer-by.

'You got me again!' the doctor would exclaim with a smile as the missile hit him or her and Hannah started to giggle.

But the one thing she didn't want to do even with Sarah was talk about her treatment. Although the play leaders had dolls with miniature drains and drips to help the children understand their treatment, the only person Hannah spoke to about it was me and as she remained in remission, her inquisitive nature began to show itself once more.

'Why are they cleaning my wiggly again, Mummy?' she'd ask as the nurses flushed out her central line which had to be done every day to ensure the site was kept completely sterile.

'To make sure there are no bugs, Han.'

'Like the bugs in my blood?'

'Different ones, but we don't want any kind of bugs to hurt you.'

She was also becoming increasingly impatient when blood was taken from her thumb on every visit to the weekly clinic where in-patients and children who were being treated for leukaemia at home were seen. Unlike the routine blood tests which were done each morning using a syringe in her central line, this one involved making a knick on the pad of her thumb with a small blade before a nurse squeezed long and hard enough to collect a few millilitres of blood. For a long time, Hannah didn't say anything about it until one day we were sitting on her bed.

'Mummy?' she asked.

'Yes, Han.'

'I've been thinking. I've got my wiggly in my chest and I know they can take blood out of that, so why do they need to use my thumb too?'

'I think it's because they need special blood from the edges of your body and not blood that's from near your heart,' I replied.

Hannah didn't say anymore but firmly refused to have a thumb test done when we next went for one.

'You can use my wiggly,' she said to the nurse as she pointed to her central line.

I knew there was no point in fighting with her because Hannah could be very sure if she made up her mind and as she remained in remission, her explanations about how she wanted things done only increased.

'Please use just a tiny bit of sticky,' Hannah would say as a nurse changed her dressings because the tape securing them irritated her skin.

'Is that enough?' she'd ask solemnly when they cut a tiny piece off the roll.

At other times Hannah would refuse to let the nurses remove all the tape securing her central line because it was just too sore.

'I think you'll have to wait until tomorrow,' she'd tell whoever had come to see her.

Or she'd agree to a dressing change but insist on helping – slowly peeling back the gauze before picking up a fresh piece and holding its edges.

'We mustn't breathe on it because there might be bugs,' she'd say to the nurse.

I knew the busy doctors and nurses might expect me to step in and stop Hannah asking so many questions and I understood that there were times when I had to draw a line with her, however sick she was. For instance, I'd told her off when a group of doctors had gathered around her bed one day and Hannah had kicked out at one as she bent down to look at her, catching her on the side of the face.

'Hannah!' I had snapped as I pushed her leg back down.

I knew that Hannah felt frustrated and angry but I had to help her learn to carry the heavy burden of being sick by sometimes imposing normal rules, however hard it felt. I'd seen for myself that many parents on the ward found it difficult to impose limits on their sick children. But while I understood how difficult it was, I didn't want Hannah to forget what normal life was like.

So I was prepared to draw lines for her on some occasions but on others I was not, and one of those was when she asked questions about what was happening. Hannah simply wanted to know about who was doing what to her, how and when and her views deserved respect. She was the one who had to live all this and while my job was to discipline her at times, it was to fight for her at others too; ask questions when necessary and ignore the answers occasionally.

I knew this because Hannah's illness had awoken a protective instinct so strong that it almost shocked me. Like any mother, I'd always felt I would do anything to protect my children. But it wasn't until my love was tested that this feeling became so fiercely practical. My need to protect her washed away my concerns about what people thought of me, the fear of doing the wrong thing and the desire to tiptoe around for fear of causing offence. Early on, I realised that I had to let go of worrying about how my actions were viewed as long as I believed they were right for Hannah.

So although medical advice was always given with the best possible intentions, there were times when I rebelled against it: 'forgetting' to brush her teeth when her mouth was bleeding during chemotherapy and too painful to disturb; or asking the nurses to wait a couple of hours so that medications, blood samples and dressing changes could be done together rather than spread out which only prolonged the discomfort.

I found my voice more and more because I wanted to make sure the quality of the life Hannah lived each day was the best it could be and if that meant making her feel safer or giving her just a few moments of respite from her pain then I would do it. Like any other parent, it was a question of balancing my child's long-term good with the short term. Sometimes that meant the rules had to be respected for Hannah's sake – but at others they had to be broken.

'She really shouldn't go into theatre with her nail varnish on,' the nurse said as she looked at me.

Hannah was getting ready to go down and have her central line changed. It was the time both of us dreaded most – she hated being put to sleep, and watching her slip into unconsciousness always made me afraid. She had to have a lumbar puncture every month for detailed blood tests to be done and we both went quiet when the time came. Hannah would be lifted onto a trolley and I'd walk beside her through the long hospital corridors – down to the nurses' station, into the lift, up one floor, out the lift, down another corridor, into another lift, down two floors, into another corridor – each step taking us nearer to theatre.

'I don't want to go to sleep,' Hannah would cry.

'It will just be for a little while,' I'd reassure her.

'But I don't want to.'

'The doctors need to make you sleepy, my darling, but it won't be for long. A nurse will be with you and I'll be there until you go to sleep.'

'But I'm not tired.'

'Well, the doctor will give you a special medicine so that you are.'

'How can he do that?'

'Because he has lots of medicines to do different things: some fight the bugs in your blood and some put you to sleep.'

For a little while Hannah would go quiet as we travelled through the hospital, but as soon as we got to the three anaesthetic rooms leading to the theatres she would start crying. Scrabbling for me with her hands, the doors would open and she would be pushed feet first into the tiny room.

'Mummy, mummy, I don't want to sleep,' she'd sob.

'I'm here,' I'd whisper. 'I'm with you.'

But as a mask was slipped over her face or the anaesthetic was connected to her central line, Hannah would struggle to stay awake even as she started falling into unconsciousness.

'Help me, help me, help me,' she would cry as her body twitched and I had to leave the room so that the staff could intubate her.

It was only when I got back into the corridor that I would start to cry. As Hannah lay unconscious in theatre, I would think of her pleas and the cries she had made as she clawed the air for me. Seeing her in pain, whether mental or physical, went against every instinct I had as a mother however much my rational self knew that she had to have treatment.

Now I looked at Hannah's toenails as the nurse held out the nail varnish remover for me and I wondered what to do. Hannah loved having her nails painted, each one a different

colour so that she could stare at the rainbow on her toes –
pink, blue, green, red, yellow – as she lay in bed. Even when
she couldn't speak, she'd wiggle her toes so the nurses could
admire them.

I knew what I had to say.

'I can't take the varnish off,' I said to the nurse.

She looked at me – sympathy and routine wrestling across
her features. Nail varnish was supposed to be removed
during a general anaesthetic so that the patient's nail bed
colour could be checked as an indicator of circulation.

'Just one?' she asked.

'No,' I replied. 'If I do a toe then you'll do a toe, then a
finger, and soon it will all come off.'

'But I think we'll have to.'

'Well, I don't want to do it. I'm sorry but I know there are
many other ways of checking that she's OK without seeing
her toenails.'

The nurse looked at me.

'If you have to take it off then I want you to do it while
she's asleep,' I said slowly. 'And if you do then I would like
someone to draw a chart with every one of her fingers and
toes written on it so that you can reapply the varnish before
she wakes up. I know it's a lot of work but it's important to
her.'

The nurse looked at me.

'We'll see what we can do,' she said with a smile.

As the nurse left the room, I looked at the colours
sparkling on Hannah's toes and breathed a sigh of relief. If I

was going to let the doctors do what they must to save my child's life, then they had to listen to me when it came to making it slightly easier for her. She loved looking at her painted nails. I wanted her to have that.

I could hear the cries as they cut through the stillness of the ward. It was the early hours of the morning and I sat up to check that Hannah was still asleep. The sobs echoed down the corridor and cut through me – a haunting lament for a son or daughter lost, an animal howl of grief that made my heart twist. Somewhere nearby, a child had lost its fight against the illness we were all trying to conquer.

These were the darkest moments on the unit – the time when my hope was stretched to its limit. Each day I clung onto it, knowing what might happen if Hannah's treatment was unsuccessful but believing it would be. Only the sight of an empty bed which hours before had been filled by a dangerously sick child, or the quiet sadness which curled around the unit when a girl or boy died, threatened to dent the dam of hope I'd built inside.

'Mummy?' I heard Hannah whisper. 'What's that noise?'

I got out of bed and sat down beside her. Looking at her pale face, I wondered how I could possibly explain what had happened without showing my fear.

'I think one of the children is very poorly and their mummy is sad,' I said softly.

'Have they died?'

Death was a concept Hannah had quickly become familiar with in hospital. It was part of life here and she knew that children who were there when she fell asleep had sometimes gone by the time she woke in the morning.

'I don't know, Han.'

I smoothed her hair back from her forehead, soft strokes to try and soothe her back into sleep. I didn't want these sounds to frighten her.

'What does heaven look like, Mummy?' she asked.

I paused for a moment. I'd tried to make death and heaven things that didn't scare Hannah when we'd talked about this before. Now she wanted to again.

'Heaven is a beautiful place where God lives,' I said. 'There are no bad people there, or medicines. Instead there are lots of apples on the trees and daisies in the fields.'

'Do you have to go to school in heaven?'

'No. You can play.'

'How do you get to heaven, Mummy?'

'If you're really, really poorly then you fall asleep and wake up there.'

'Will I go to heaven?'

'Not now, Han. You only go when you're very, very sick.'

'I'm not poorly enough?'

I paused for a moment. A sadness so strong filled me that I could hardly breathe but at the same time I felt a sliver of still peacefulness – gratitude that Hannah could ask questions and trust me to give her any answers I could.

'No, darling. You're not poorly enough and I promise that you'll wake up tomorrow for a whole new day.'

I bent to kiss her.

'Now close your eyes and I'll stay right beside you.'

I pulled Hannah's duvet around her and waited until I was sure she was sleeping again. My body felt tense, my skin almost prickling, as if an aftershock of the woman's cries still pulsed through me. I thought of all the other parents here in this huge hospital, wondering who else had lost their child tonight. If it wasn't now, it would be tomorrow or the next day; if it wasn't an illness, it would be a child brought in after a terrible accident. I shivered as I thought of those parents for whom bereavement came in an instant, the mothers and fathers who had no sign that grief was about to rip a hole in the fabric of their life. Even though I had watched Hannah walk a road I had wished many times that I could travel for her, I was glad I had been given the chance to walk by her side.

She and I had had time together – to talk, smile, play games and just lie in silence. I'd had time to comfort and soothe her, prepare her in whatever way I could for whatever lay ahead and give thanks for being her mother. Now I thought of other mothers suffering a pain I couldn't even begin to imagine as they tried to negotiate a world they never wanted to know and vowed that I would never take time for granted again. As I listened to the steady breathing of

Hannah's sleep, I knew that once again she'd taught me just how much I had to be thankful for.

CHAPTER THREE

Not Ours to Keep

❁

It's Easter 2009 and I've just got back from holiday. It was brilliant. We went to Cornwall for a week and I really enjoyed myself because there have been loads of times in the past when I haven't got to go away with Dad, Oli, Lucy and Phoebe during the school holidays. I went last year but didn't enjoy it much because I was ill so I spent most of the time in my wheelchair and kept getting cold, which meant Mum had to put me back in the car with a rug. We spent ages sitting in there together while the others did stuff, which really annoyed me.

But this time I felt much better and wondered what my doctors would say if they could see me playing on the arcade machines and eating candyfloss. You see they thought I wasn't going to get any better when I left hospital nearly two years ago after saying no to a transplant. I knew that not having the operation would limit my life but I just didn't want to have it. Instead I was given a pacemaker, and although my heart still doesn't work properly and I have to spend a lot of time in bed, I'm stronger now and no one expected that. I like the fact that I've proved the doctors wrong. I did it the first time when I was little and had leukaemia. Now I'm doing it again. I don't know if I'll be so lucky a third time, but I bet those doctors are amazed I've made it this far.

We left Mum at home so that she could have a rest while we went to Cornwall. With all of us, the animals and the horses, she gets pretty tired so she wanted to be by herself for a bit. But it didn't work out like that because my great aunt Kitty got ill as soon as we left so she came to stay and Mum didn't have the holiday for herself that she'd planned. But she didn't mind because that's just how she is. If anyone gets sick, then she's the person who looks after them.

If you ask me it was brave of Dad to take us all away on his own, though. Oli, Lucy and I can look after ourselves most of the time but you have to keep an eye on Phoebe, which is hard because she never stops and Dad's not used to it like Mum is. We stayed in a caravan in a town called Looe and went to the arcades, played bingo, ate fish and chips and even went gold panning in a river. I found a tiny chip but not enough to make a ring or anything.

Dad also took us shopping and bought me a purple and red checked jacket with a furry hood and a pair of boots for Phoebe. But she didn't want to let go of them after Dad had paid and the girl in the shop needed to put them in a bag. So I had to chase her around the shop because I knew someone might think we'd stolen the boots if we walked out without a bag. That's what I mean – Phoebe is a terror.

I was a bit worried before we went away because my wheel-chair didn't fit in the back of the car. But I was also happy we weren't taking it because although it's pink which means it's as nice as it can be, I still like to walk. I shouldn't have worried, though, because I didn't need my chair in the end. That's what seems to happen when I'm really excited about something – somehow I find the energy to do it. It's only afterwards that I feel ill.

I think that's why I managed to go on a rollercoaster in Cornwall. I really wanted to do it because I'd never been on one before. But as we queued, we saw a sign which said, 'Don't go on if you've got a heart complaint,' and I felt worried that Dad was going to stop me from going on. But then he smiled and said we wouldn't tell Mum so I knew he was going to let me. It was amazing. Flying through the air and laughing as the wind rushed by. It was so fast. I screamed my head off.

Now I'm home again but I'm still not back at school. I've been trying to go for months but it hasn't gone that well because I've been ill or something else has happened and I'm missing my mates. Simone's been telling me what's going on and the latest news is that she and Tiago have split up. I don't think she's that bothered about it.

I wish I could be at school, though, instead of hearing about it on the phone and one of the reasons why I like being with my friends is because they don't look at me all worried or go quiet as they wonder if I'm tiring myself out. They know that if I've done too much the colour will drain from my face, I'll see spots in front of my eyes and have to lie down until I pick back up again. They trust me to know when I need to slow down and leave me to get on with it, which is what I really like.

But since I came out of hospital after having the pacemaker I haven't been able to get to proper school a lot of the time. Instead I go to the one at Hereford Hospital where the day only lasts the morning and we have our lessons in a classroom at the end of the children's ward. There are usually four pupils and two teachers, which is great because I get help with maths which is my hardest subject. I don't get numbers and my mind wanders easily when I don't understand something so I usually end up staring out of the window. But it's not so easy to daydream when you've got a teacher sitting right next to you.

I like going to hospital school, though, because at least it means I'm well enough to do something. When I first came out of hospital nearly two years ago, after saying no to the transplant, I just lay in bed all the time because I was so ill that the doctors had said I wouldn't get any better. But I knew I would, even though my heart wouldn't, if you see what I mean. I had the pacemaker and a drug called Dobutamine to make my heart beat stronger. Most of all, I knew I'd get well because I hate being in hospital so much that being at home always makes me feel better.

The Dobutamine gave me really bad headaches, though, and was a real pain because I had to have it through a central line attached to a syringe driver that went everywhere I did. It was like Hansel and Gretel but with a syringe driver instead of bread. So even though it kept me going, I was really happy when I stopped taking the Dobutamine last year and I've been getting stronger ever since. At the moment I seem to be doing OK with just my pacemaker.

I know exactly where it is because it's underneath a scar on my chest, just across from my heart. It's got four wires, one going into each chamber of my heart, and sometimes I can feel it zapping. The worst, though, is having it tested because when one side of the pacemaker is switched off, I can feel my heart beating really hard against my chest until they turn it back on and I can feel the difference immediately.

Most of the time, the problems with my heart mean that I just have to make sure I don't get too tired because that's how a bad heart makes you feel – so tired you can't even lift your head off the pillow sometimes. It's because there are four chambers in everyone's heart – two on the left and two on the right – and the ones on the right side of mine don't work properly. Think of it like doors that are blowing in the wind instead of being locked shut. The blood in my heart does not pump properly so my heart needs all my energy to keep going, which doesn't leave much for the rest of me.

The pacemaker has helped, though, because if my heart gets tired and slow it says, 'Jump to it.' My heart can also beat too fast and the pacemaker slows it down as well. It's a bit like a schoolteacher telling the class to sit still and start working. Occasionally I can feel it when I'm ill in bed and my blood pressure has dropped. Sometimes it's like a vibration but at others it's more like a ping! I know it's the pacemaker because before I had it fitted I never felt like that. Sometimes it stops me going to sleep but most of the time I can't feel it.

The doctors know what's going on in my heart because they do scans like the ones women have when they're pregnant.

They're weird because I can see my heart and the blood going in and out of it in different colours on the screen – red and blue. That's when I can see the valves aren't closing properly and one of the sides of my heart is leaking which I know isn't good. Even though I feel better now, the doctors have told me my heart has not improved, which upsets me a bit because I think I've been doing OK.

Now we're back home after our holiday and Oli, Lucy and Phoebe have started school again, which means the house is quiet. I get lonely sometimes because there aren't many other ill children around here so there's no one of my age to talk to. But I also quite like being quiet because although I love my brother and sisters, they can really annoy me at times too. Oli and Lucy know all the best hiding places in my bedroom so if I try to keep something secret they'll always find it. Phoebe is also in and out all the time and if I'm feeling tired I just want her to leave me alone even though I know she doesn't understand. When I'm really ill it's as much as Mum can do to get her to come down the stairs in the morning without screaming, and so it's not surprising that she doesn't get it when I'm just ordinary ill.

Being on my own again means I've got lots of time to think and I've been wondering why people are still so interested about me not having the transplant. Sometimes I get sick of talking about it because I think there are other more important things to say. But everyone went mad when they found out about my decision after a newspaper did a story about it. That was last year but journalists still ring up to see how I am and ask the same things over and over again. Why didn't you have the transplant? What made you decide not to? Will you reconsider? One even asked me once how I wanted my funeral to be. Questions like that annoy me. I'm thirteen and I've had to talk about dying. It's not that I hate mentioning it but I don't like going on about it. No one does. I can talk about it to a certain extent but then I go quiet.

I just wish people would accept that I don't want the transplant. I want to be at home even though I know the doctors have said I won't get better. It was a big decision but I wanted to make it even though I felt scared and sad and anxious all at the same time. Mum and Dad said they'd choose for me if I wanted them to but I didn't because I knew they might feel guilty if something went wrong. It was my decision. No one else's. And I made it for the right reasons.

Now the summer term at school has started, I'm looking forward to September because I hope I'll be well enough to start Year 10. It's scary because it only seems like yesterday that I was in Year 7. I've already picked my GCSEs and I'm doing the five main subjects plus ICT and something else I can't remember. I'm trying to do a bit of everything because I'm at a crossroads about jobs and need to learn as many different things as I can. At the moment there are three jobs I'd like to do: mostly I want to be like Cheryl Cole but I also want to be a fashion designer and make pink clothes because there aren't enough of them, or be the boss of a company like Alan Sugar in *The Apprentice* – really rich and in charge of everyone.

To keep myself lazy busy now I'm home and everyone else is back at school, I've been watching my new favourite film –

Mamma Mia! It's brilliant, cool and fab all at the same time. I like the dancing and the jokes but most of all I love the singing and can't decide which is my favourite song. It's great when the lady sings 'Does Your Mother Know' to her boyfriend on the beach, but I also like 'Honey Honey' because it always makes me laugh when Sophie sings 'You're a doggone beast' and giggles.

The songs are cool and I've been sitting in my room reading the words on the CD cover and singing along. Sometimes I get up and dance a bit too. Head banging is my favourite thing because it makes me feel dizzy, although I sometimes have to sit down if I do too much. But it feels great while I'm doing it, and that's what counts, isn't it?

Of all the systems, processes and cycles that make up the miracle of human life, perhaps the most amazing is the heart – the power house of the human body which keeps the brain and organs fed with blood. An adult heart beats on average between 60 and 100 times every minute of every hour, day, week, month and year of a person's life, however long – a feat of natural engineering that has never been surpassed by the bridges, rockets or machines built by people.

Since New Year we'd known Hannah's heart wasn't pumping as effectively as it should have been. But as time had passed it had become increasingly clear that the problems were not being solved by medication. Hannah was still tired, weak and out of breath – the classic symptoms of heart abnormalities – and I was terrified when the doctors told me she was suffering mild heart failure. I tried to stem my panic by telling myself the term was a catch-all which covered a huge range of possibilities from sudden, severe and fatal heart failure to temporary symptoms from which a patient can recover. Heart failure can mean anything from a weakening of the muscles of the heart to a virus which disrupts its electrical signals or a glitch in one of the valves. No one knew what was causing Hannah's problems and I simply didn't dare consider they might be anything other than temporary.

But as she rested after her second round of chemotherapy, Dr Williams and her cardiologist Dr Wright decided they needed to do a more in-depth scan to give them a fuller picture of what was happening. Hannah had had scans including ECGs to measure the electrical activity of her heart and mini echocardiograms which used sound waves to create a picture of it, but now the doctors needed to know more.

'Is my heart still poorly, Mummy?' Hannah had asked when I told her she was going to have a special X-ray.

'The doctors aren't sure so they want to look very closely,' I told her.

'Has my heart got bugs like my blood?'

'We don't think so, but Dr Wright will use his special machine to find out.'

'Will he make my heart better?'

'I hope so, Han.'

A couple of days later we were taken to the X-ray unit, where Hannah lay on a bed as Dr Wright smeared gel onto her chest before pushing a probe across it. Working around the central line coming out of her chest, he guided it until a picture appeared on the monitor beside Hannah's bed.

Before now the scans had only contained blurry outlines and shadows but this one was giving us a far more concrete image of what was happening inside Hannah's body. Andrew stood close to me as we watched her heart expanding and contracting, the blood rushing in and out of it in waves of blue and red across the screen.

Pressing buttons as he moved the probe across Hannah's chest, Dr Wright freeze-framed images to take detailed measurements. Lines and shapes, trapezoids and rectangles appeared on the images to give an exact assessment of Hannah's heart rate and function. Numbers popped up on the screen and I stared at them, willing the figures to give us good news, praying that it wouldn't be bad.

When the scan was over the doctors went away to talk before calling Andrew and me back to see them. Their faces were serious as we sat down.

'I'm afraid the results were not what we'd hoped,' Dr Wright told us and for a moment I wanted to turn and run, not allow myself to hear another word of what he was about to say.

'The valves on the left-hand side of Hannah's heart are working perfectly but the ones on the right are not doing so well,' Dr Wright continued. 'The entire muscle of her heart is also working at a decreased output.'

'What do you mean?' Andrew asked, his voice strained with fear.

'The scan has shown that Hannah has cardiomyopathy,' Dr Wright told us. 'This means that the muscles of her heart are damaged, and she also has problems with her fractional shortening, which is the amount her heart expands and contracts with each beat. The bigger it is, the better the heart is pumping, but I'm afraid we've discovered that Hannah's heart function is low.'

Andrew stared at the doctors intently as I sat without saying a word, unable to take it all in, hardly hearing what was being said.

'How low?' Andrew asked softly.

'Seventeen per cent.'

He slumped back in his chair, stunned as I tried to understand. Seventeen out of a possible hundred? Hannah's heart was struggling to beat at less than a fifth of the capacity of a healthy child's? I wanted to scream, to drown out the roar inside me. How could Hannah have another enemy to fight? How unfair could one life be? I shivered as rage pulsed up inside me, knowing that pain was close behind it.

'I understand that this is sudden news for you both but there is a lot of medication we can give Hannah to help her body cope with this,' Dr Williams said gently. 'There are drugs to combat fluid retention and others to make her heart beat more efficiently or increase her blood pressure.'

'But she will get better?' Andrew cried.

Dr Williams paused for a moment.

'This is a very rare situation which happens in only a tiny percentage of children who undergo chemotherapy,' he said carefully. 'And I'm afraid we just can't be sure what will happen to Hannah's heart in the future. It is possible that new muscle will grow with her as she gets older and her heart function will improve, but we cannot say for certain.'

'But what caused this?' I said at last, the words feeling thick in my mouth as I spoke them.

'We think Hannah has had a very rare reaction to the chemotherapy and the drugs given to combat the leukaemia have damaged the muscles to her heart,' Dr Williams replied. 'Cases like this are very, very rare but we think this is what has happened to Hannah.'

Coldness flooded through my body. The medicine that was saving Hannah's life might also be harming it.

There was another storm approaching.

'As you know, we would usually complete all six courses of chemotherapy to maximise Hannah's chances of continuing in long-term remission from the leukaemia,' Dr Williams said. 'But given that we believe the chemotherapy is responsible, it means there is a risk of further damage to her heart if we continue Hannah's treatment. I'm afraid we just cannot be sure.'

Memories of the notes and information leaflets we'd been given rushed through my head. Line after line of side effects and possibilities – one-in-a-million chances that we hadn't been able to consider as Hannah's life hung in the balance.

'What do you mean?' Andrew cried. 'Does that mean Hannah has to stop treatment?'

'Not necessarily, but the problems with her heart are serious enough for us to think that if she does have another round of chemotherapy, it should be her last,' Dr Williams replied. 'We do not want to run the risk of causing further and catastrophic damage.'

Everyone was silent. How could Hannah stop her chemo now? She had only completed two cycles and we'd always been told she needed six to maximise her chances of beating the cancer for ever. How could we deny her that? How could we forgo her best possible chance of defeating her illness? I thought of the blood cells deep inside her, the unknown trigger that had caused them to malfunction. If she did not complete her chemotherapy then surely it might happen again? I couldn't bear the thought. But how could we risk further damage being done to her heart? Panic filled me as I wondered how we would ever make this decision.

'You will need to decide quickly what you want to do because Hannah is due to start treatment again in a few days,' Dr Williams continued quietly.

I knew he had children about Hannah's age. He was a parent just like Andrew and I.

'What would you do?' I asked, silently begging him to give me the answer that I wasn't sure I could find myself.

'I'm afraid I can't tell you,' Dr Wright replied softly. 'This really is a decision that only you can make.'

Fear filled me as I heard those words. How could Andrew and I decide to stop the treatment that was meant to be saving

Hannah's life? But how could we continue the chemotherapy knowing we might risk Hannah's health in another way? Surely it was an impossible choice?

Only one thing was clear to me: we had to speak to Hannah. She was the person at the centre of this, the one who would be affected by whatever we decided for her, and in the depths of my uncertainty I knew we must talk to her. I had explained every step of Hannah's treatment to her and felt she had been a lot calmer because of it. Now we would talk to her again because although the decision about whether to continue with the chemotherapy or not belonged solely to Andrew and me, I wanted Hannah to understand what was happening.

Many parents on the ward were careful about how much they told their children for fear of scaring them, and before Hannah fell ill I would probably have done the same. But I'd learned that children who have felt death whisper at the edges of their world can become wise beyond their years. Even at such a young age, Hannah was completely attuned to her treatment: she knew if her drugs were too early or late and was also very aware of being different because she had a heart monitor.

'I'm the only one with this, aren't I, Mummy?' she'd say after looking around at the other children on the ward. 'Why do I have one and not the others?'

'Because your heart is poorly and the doctors need to listen to it all the time.'

'What does it say?'

'It doesn't say anything. Instead it beats.'

'What does that sound like?'

'A bit like a train. Bo-boom, bo-boom, bo-boom. The noises tell the doctors what your heart is doing.'

'A bit like when I'm playing with Oli and you hear us shouting so you come to see us?'

'Yes, Han. A bit like that.'

I didn't mind that we did things differently with Hannah because it felt right – just as it did with Andrew. While many parents moved onto the oncology ward together with their children, he and I had had very separate roles from the moment Hannah was admitted to hospital – my place was with her while he was at home with Oli and Lucy. I missed him terribly and there were nights when I felt so alone without him. But we spoke every evening and Andrew visited often. His calm presence always comforted me but so did the thought that he was at home with Oli and Lucy. It meant normal life was continuing and reminded me that Hannah and I had something to go back to.

Now Andrew and I had an important decision to make and the doctors, who had always supported our decision to include Hannah in conversations, agreed to speak to her with us.

We walked to Hannah's room where we gathered around her bed and I sat down beside her.

'Dr Williams wants to talk to you, Han,' I said softly as I stroked her feet. 'He thinks that if you have more medicine to kill the leukaemia bugs then your heart might get more poorly. But if you don't have more then the leukaemia bugs might grow bigger and we wouldn't want that. Mummy and Daddy have to decide whether to give you more medicine.'

She looked up at me.

'I don't want any more,' she said.

'I know they're horrible Han,' I said slowly. 'But the medicines are killing the bugs in your blood and the doctors will make sure they don't hurt too much when you have them again.'

'But they do hurt,' she cried.

'I know, but we all want you to get better.'

Hannah looked at Dr Williams and we waited for her to speak. I wished I knew what was happening inside her, understood completely all that she thought and felt.

'I'll have to think about it,' she said at last.

~

Hannah was wrapped up against the cold as she sat in the wheelchair. She was wearing a soft cotton top with buttons down the front and the tubes leading to her central line spilled out of it. To stop them pulling, they'd been put into a 'wiggly' bag which hung on a satin ribbon around her neck. The strap on the small material bag was padded with pieces of foam that I'd stitched on because Hannah was still so thin everything had to be soft or padded to make it comfortable on her skin.

A drip bag was clamped to one side of the wheelchair and a syringe driver to the other. The box measured about six inches by eight and contained syringes which pumped Hannah's medications into her bloodstream at one mil every hour. She was wearing a fleece jacket with a fur-lined hood and three rugs were wrapped around her legs to protect her from the February chill because we were going to high mass at Birmingham's Catholic cathedral St Chad's. It was very close to the children's hospital and I wanted to take Hannah out now that she was in the rest period before her third round of chemotherapy started.

A calm clarity had filled me after my initial rush of fear about our decision. As my anger and sadness had calmed a little, I'd realised that the choice Andrew and I had to make wasn't a question of right or wrong because we couldn't be sure whatever path we chose to take. All we knew for certain was that the less chemo Hannah had, the more likely the leukaemia was to return and we had to weigh that against the possible effects on her heart, which were an unknown. And so we'd decided to give Hannah one final round of chemotherapy – knowing it would be her last. One last chance at making sure the cancer didn't return.

'I'm tired of being in hospital, Mummy,' Hannah had said as she lay in bed after we'd spoken to Dr Williams. 'I want to go home.'

The more time we spent in hospital, the more regularly Hannah asked for this now and it worried me that her longing for home might make her resistant to more treatment. I knew I would somehow have to convince her to accept our decision if she was but didn't want to have to. The chemotherapy was enough of a burden without forcing Hannah to have it against her will.

'I want you to go home too,' I said as I sat beside her. 'And we will as soon as the doctors have given you all your medicines. But we have to make sure the bugs in your blood are really gone first.'

We didn't talk any more about it until the next morning when Dr Williams came back to see us. After he'd examined

Hannah and checked her charts, she'd looked at him with a serious face.

'I have decided that I will have some more medicine,' she said solemnly.

Dr Williams turned to me.

'Is this what Mum thinks too?' he asked.

'Yes,' I said.

'We'll start again next week.'

All we could do was inch forward, hoping that we had made the right choice, and I thought about it for the thousandth time now as I stopped to tuck the rugs more closely around Hannah's legs and a picture of Andrew, Oli and Lucy flashed into my head. Was Andrew bending to wipe Oli's hands now? Or feeding Lucy her lunch? Sometimes it felt as if the life we'd all lived together was so far away we might never get back to it. Hannah and I had slipped so completely into the rhythm of hospital life that it was a shock when I'd first left the building and the real world had burst in again. A wall of sound had surrounded me – sirens wailing, people shouting and cars beeping their horns – as I dashed out to buy food at the supermarket or visit the dental hospital to have treatment for the increasingly bad toothache I was getting.

'What kind of food do you eat?' the dentist had asked me when I first saw him. 'Do you smoke? Are you under a lot of stress?'

When I'd told him that Hannah was in hospital being treated for leukaemia, his voice had softened as he'd said that intense stress could weaken teeth. After having root canal treatment and two veneers fitted, I hoped the problems were at an end.

Now I walked towards the cathedral entrance and wondered how Hannah felt to be outside again. Apart from the visit home for Oli's birthday, she had only glimpsed the world when I'd pushed her to the front door of the hospital to smell the fresh air. I knew it must be strange for her now and pushed a little harder to get us more quickly into the quiet of the cathedral where we sat down near the altar – me on the end of a pew and Hannah in her chair in the aisle beside me. An organ played softly as we waited for mass to start and the hush of the cathedral surrounded us. The peace and quiet was one of the main reasons why I enjoyed going to church so much – it gave me a chance to reflect, which always soothed me.

As a child, my grandmother had taken me to mass every Sunday during term time, and on weekdays as well in the holidays. But as a teenager, I'd rebelled and stopped going so much before life and work had taken over and I hadn't attended church because I was simply too busy. But I'd begun to go again after having children because I wanted them to grow up with a faith just as I had done. Although I was a Catholic, it didn't matter to me what kind of church we went to – Baptist or Methodist, Protestant or Catholic – I just liked the stillness of any place of worship.

But now as I sat with Hannah, the questions crowded into my mind. Had Andrew and I made the right decision about continuing with the chemotherapy? Were we giving Hannah a better chance at life? Or were we harming her? Was it even right to put her through any of this at all? Sometimes it seemed like madness that the effects of a hoped-for cure seemed as painful as those of the disease and however much I knew Hannah needed treatment, guilt filled me when I thought of the suffering it caused her.

The priest's words washed over me as he started to recite the mass and I drunk in the stillness of the cathedral, letting it take root inside. I would need all the strength my faith could give me for the next stage of our journey and for Hannah's sake I must believe completely in the decision Andrew and I had made. We had done what we thought was right which was all we could do.

Hannah would start chemotherapy again next week and there were no guarantees. No one could tell us whether we would be thankful or regretful of our decision in the future because we could not know what was to come. But one thing was certain: Hannah needed our strength and we had to trust in the choice we'd made for her. Our faith was the least she deserved.

Once again Hannah's immune system was reduced to almost nothing as the chemotherapy drove her white blood cell counts down to stop her immune system attacking the drugs. As they fed into her system, I counted down the days until the most intensive phase ended, knowing this would be the last time her body could latch onto the possibility of the long-term recovery that chemotherapy offered. I hoped and prayed it would do its job well.

Because of her heart problems, Hannah could no longer have regular lumbar punctures to check that she was still in remission. Instead her blood was taken and sent to Italy where highly specialised tests were run on it. It took two weeks to get the results back and it was an anxious time as we waited. But just as she'd done after the previous two chemo cycles, Hannah recovered amazingly quickly and started growing stronger as her blood counts rose days after the intensive phase of drugs ended. Soon we learned that she was still free from cancer and a rush of gratitude filled me. Her heart had also stayed the same during this treatment cycle and we knew we were lucky that it had not worsened.

As Hannah's health improved, I tried to take her out of her room in the high dependency unit a little more and we made trips around the hospital to go to the café or see a man who brought snakes and spiders in for the children to look at. Hannah was handed a snake to hold as she sat in her chair, and although we had to go back to her bed twenty minutes later I was amazed she was strong enough to leave it when she'd only recently been so weak.

But I wanted to get her out and about a little more because now Hannah's chemotherapy had come to an end it was only a matter of time before she left hospital. She would be discharged as soon as her blood counts were high enough and the doctors were sure she was free of infections. Then we would go home to see what the future held.

My excitement about returning to normal life had been tinged with fear, though, after an overnight trip home showed me just how difficult it might be. I went because Oli in particular was missing me and I wanted to tell him that I'd soon be back. After almost three months away I was longing to see Andrew and the children but it was the first time I'd left Hannah for any real length of time and I felt suddenly anxious as I got on the train home. I couldn't stop thinking of her. I knew she would be well looked after, but what about all the tiny things that only I knew? Like the way her duvet had to be smooth on the bed or the fact that she liked a few toys but not too many on her feet?

Anger suddenly flared inside me as I thought about it sitting in a carriage surrounded by ordinary people travelling on an ordinary day. For them today bled into yesterday and tomorrow, another in a succession of peacefully average days. They didn't know how my hands itched to pull the emergency cord, how every beat of the train on the tracks pulsed into me – each taking me further away from Hannah. I shouldn't have left her, I should be with her now just as I'd been since the day she went into hospital. I felt so confused as I watched houses and trees rush by. How could I feel so desperate that my journey was taking me away from Hannah when it was also bringing me nearer to Oli and Lucy?

When the train finally pulled into the station, I got off and walked to a long flight of steps that would take me to the car park. Looking down, I saw Andrew coming up with Oli and Lucy. The children smiled and shrieked as they saw me. Lucy was wearing her favourite pink fairy outfit with a crown on her head and Oli was in shorts even though it was only early March. A rush of love filled me as I ran down the steps towards them. I'd done the right thing by coming home. I'd missed them so much and their smiles told me I was right to be here.

But almost as soon as I scooped them into my arms, doubt seeped over the edges of my joy. Even as I was reunited with one part of myself, I felt as if I'd left another behind, and wondered how I was going to reconcile them when we got home because Hannah's needs were so different to Oli and Lucy's – on oxygen twenty-four hours a day, she still wasn't eating, her feed had to be administered by a nasogastric tube and her drug regime was also very complicated.

All I could do was put my worries to one side and draw on what Hannah had already taught me in the weeks, months and years ahead. What had happened to her wasn't about guilt, blame, bad luck or mistakes. I couldn't control her future – her life, death or recovery – because Hannah wasn't an object I owned to succeed or fail with. She had been given to Andrew and me because we were strong enough to be her guardians and we would love and protect her, just as we would Oli and Lucy.

All Hannah wanted was to leave hospital and so I urged the doctors to release us as soon as possible. At first, they weren't keen to let us go, but they soon realised that my will was as strong as my daughter's when I really wanted something. Hannah hated it in hospital and I felt sure she would get stronger once we left. It just seemed logical to me that the happier she was, the healthier she would be.

I remembered the moment she was born, the feeling of the tears slipping salty down the side of my face as I held Hannah for the first time. Back then I'd known how lucky I was to have her after waiting for so long. But it was only now I knew for certain that she was not mine to keep or lose: Hannah, like every child, was a gift, not a right. I must cherish her for as long as she was mine.

CHAPTER FOUR

Look for the Love

❀

I've been in bed for a few days because I went to a horse show last weekend and it flattened me. I wasn't feeling that well before I went but going really knocked it out of me. I knew Mum and Dad were worried but I don't get to visit horse shows often so I really wanted to go. For ages after my heart got worse there was no chance of me being able to because it was too cold for me during the winter and I wasn't well enough. But it's spring now, I'm stronger and Lucy is such a good rider that her bedroom is covered in rosettes and I want to see her win some for myself.

'We'll see how you feel nearer the time,' Mum kept telling me when I asked about it.

I tried to be extra bouncy to show her I was well enough even though it didn't make a huge difference. It's a bit like salt and vinegar crisps and sea salt and balsamic vinegar crisps – the tastes are a tiny bit different but they're the same really. That's what it's like when I try to be bouncy – I get a bit more energy but not so much anyone would really notice. It's not like I can suddenly turn into Zebedee or something.

But I did the best I could and Lucy and I got more and more excited as the time to leave for the show got closer. She was going to ride Mr Minty, who is a grey which means his coat is white, and another pony she'd been lent to ride. His name is Gunner and he's a bit more delicate than Mr Minty, who's chunky. Gunner is brown with white socks and a white blaze on his nose. He was too much of a handful for the little girl who had him before so her parents lent him to Lucy because she's not afraid of anything.

We counted down the days until the one before we were due to leave when Mum drove the horse lorry from the garage where it's kept and parked it outside our house. Some horse lorries are massive, with room for six horses and lots of people. Ours is more of a van really but we still call it a lorry because that's the proper name. It's old but there's room in the front for three people to sit next to the driver. Behind is a living area with a tiny kitchen, a big bed on a platform above the driver's seat that you have to climb up a ladder to get to and a door through to the horses at the back.

As soon as the lorry arrived, I got in and started asking Lucy to go and get everything we needed from the house – duvets and pillows, food and drinks. But although I still didn't know what Mum was thinking, I knew she must be coming round when I saw her put my medicine box and oxygen cylinder into the van. Then when everything was finally ready, she told me I could go and I jumped up and down because I was so happy. After that I went to hide my new gold sandals under the bed because although Lucy's not that fussed by them and she was going to be away with me anyway, I couldn't be sure about Phoebe. She likes going into my room and taking my things when I'm not there so I hid my sandals because they're my favourite thing.

We left early on Friday morning and the journey took so long that I felt really tired by the time we arrived and couldn't get up the ladder to bed. Luckily we'd brought a camp bed for Mum so I went on that and she went up top with Lucy. The next morning I stayed in bed late before Mum put me in our friend Tina's lorry to watch the riding. It's heated in there and much better than being outside because my circulation is bad and I feel ill if I get too cold. So I sat in the van which was parked right next to the arena and watched the jumping from there. Lucy was great. She looked really smart in her white shirt, blue jacket, gloves and boots. She's supposed to wear a hair net but most of the time she just ties her hair up and puts it in her hat because she prefers it that way.

I stayed in Tina's lorry until the jumping was over and then went back to ours where Mum covered me in blankets and duvets to warm me up because I'd still managed to get cold even in the warm lorry. But just as I was trying to go to sleep, a karaoke started somewhere and it felt as if the people were singing right next to our van. Then the lorry started shaking because of the wind and that's when I got a bit cross, which I do sometimes when I feel really ill. I don't think anyone can be cheerful all the time if they feel really bad. Mum gave me a pill to help me sleep, though, and I got up again late on the Sunday before going back to Tina's lorry to watch the jumping.

Lucy ended up winning two classes, coming second in two and fourth in one. She pretended to be pleased but I knew she wanted to win them all really. Then we left the show and although I was tired by the time we got home on Sunday night, I was still glad I'd been. I'd enjoyed getting excited before it and now I was enjoying being excited knowing I'd gone. The horse show was an adventure and I don't get too many of those.

I learned about adventures from the *Famous Five* books. I know they're for little kids and there's some stuff like that which I don't like – don't go there with *Hannah Montana* because it's stupid. But I've always remembered the *Famous Five* because the children do exciting things like going exploring or camping outside at night. They're much better than the Secret Seven, who just sit in their shed all the time. Weirdly, there are only four *Famous Five* children – Julian, Dick and Anne, who are brothers and sister, and George, who is a tomboy. That's because the fifth member of their group is George's dog Timmy, who goes everywhere with them. I'm not sure that Ted would go with me if I had an adventure, but it would be good if he did.

The Famous Five's adventures happen in the school holidays when Julian, Dick and Anne go to stay with George in her house beside the sea. My favourite one is called *Five Run Away Together* when the children leave home because George's mum is in hospital and the lady looking after them is horrible. So they take lots of food from the cupboards, sail to an island in George's boat and stay there until they find out that the nasty woman is even nastier than they thought because she's kidnapped a little girl. So the Famous Five tell the police who arrest the woman and the children go back to the island for more adventures until George's mother gets home.

I like the way the Famous Five are always looking for adventures even when they're told not to, and I wish I could do what they do – live in a cottage by the sea and not care about anything. If I could go on an adventure, I'd be like the Famous Five or maybe the kids in M.I.9. They're in a TV programme called *M.I. High* and they're secret agents who spend their time trying to catch baddies.

I've only had one real adventure but didn't even realise I was having it until it was over. It happened when I was in hospital after my heart got bad, but it was only when I got home and had the chance to think about everything that I realised I'd had it. I'd seen so many different things on the ward, had X-rays taken and drains put in. I'd even had a pacemaker fitted, which is quite unusual for someone as young as me.

To be honest, I didn't enjoy my adventure too much, though, so I'd like to have another by flying around the world to see the Eiffel Tower, the Leaning Tower of Pisa and the Statue of Liberty. I also want to go to China and see how different chow mein tastes there, find out what coffee is like in Brazil and eat pasta in Italy. Then I'd go to Australia to find out just how tall the roof of the Sydney Opera House is. I'm not sure about Africa because I think it might be too hot for me but I'd like to go on safari. I could go to the West Midlands Safari Park, I suppose, but it's not the same.

I think quite a lot about what I'd really like to do and the places I'd like to go. Maybe I do it more than other kids my age because I'm different to them. I can't do as much and sometimes I feel wise compared to them because I've had experiences most children haven't had. Don't get me wrong, I don't see my friends as more or less than me and it feels as if we're all the same when I'm with them. I want them to see me as a regular teenager with nothing wrong. But I know some people don't and that's why I wish sometimes that I could be normal and all this would go away.

The main thing that makes me different is that I've had to think about dying sometimes. But I've learned to push those kinds of thoughts away because it's no good keeping them in my head. Mostly I manage to, but it's hard if I've been very ill. That doesn't happen often but sometimes my heart can get suddenly worse and I'm so poorly that I can't really remember what's happened when I get better a few days later. That's when I feel very scared and the thoughts are rocks in my head because I wonder why there weren't more signs before I got really ill. And if I didn't think I was too bad when my heart was getting worse then maybe I'm sicker than I think right now?

But then I tell myself that everybody feels as if they're going to die when they get ill and I know I'm not going to today: I've had an infection and it's cleared up so I'm fine again. At times like those I make myself think about something else so I read a book, go on the computer or watch TV. There's no point wasting time feeling bad and so I remind myself about all the good things there are, like:

NATURE: I like water because otherwise there'd be nothing to drink; my animals like my cat, dog, chickens and hamster (I also like fish because you can eat them and keep them in a tank as well); I like red and pink roses, the blue climber that was at the bottom of the garden in our old house, summer when it's hot but not too hot and winter because I like snow even though it makes my fingers go numb.

FOOD: There are loads I like but some are chocolate, watermelon, spaghetti bolognaise, Sunday roasts, salami, tortilla chips, sausage rolls and pork pies. I also love Dad's stew so much that once I had two bowlfuls, followed by a big plate of tiramisu, and had to go to hospital when I got a pain in my chest which blooming well hurt. After doing loads of tests, the doctors told us it was only indigestion and I think Dad felt a bit bad about giving me so much to eat, but I was the one who'd asked for second helpings.

MUSIC: *High School Musical,* obviously; The Saturdays; *Love Machine* by Girls Aloud; Cheryl Cole because she does *The X Factor* and you can tell she's pretty even when she's got too much makeup on; and ABBA.

SMELLS: Moroccan Rose shower gel from the Body Shop is lovely, and I also like the Ocean candle from there too. Gwen Stefani's perfume is nice, and I've got another one called Top Model which I like. Dad's stew would also have to be one of my favourite smells – even if it did make everyone think I was really ill.

Oli and Lucy giggled with delight as I spread out huge white sheets of paper on the living-room floor, tucking them under the sofa to make sure everything was covered. The red carpet disappeared as the floor became a sea of white with five margarine tubs full of brightly coloured paint sitting in the middle.

'Can we start, Mummy?' Oli asked as Lucy tottered towards the tubs.

I nodded as he plunged his fingers into the paint – blue first and then yellow, the colours smearing together on his skin.

'Squoosh hard, Oli,' I urged as he pressed his hands onto the paper.

He laughed as he stared at the two mottled prints he'd made, and I grabbed Lucy.

'How about one at a time?' I laughed as she thrust her hands into every colour.

Hannah was watching us from one end of the sofa where she sat with her drip stand beside her.

'Why don't you have a go too?' I asked as I let go of Lucy and crawled across the paper to put two tubs of paint at Hannah's feet.

She bent forward slowly, dipping her fingers into green and red before leaning down. As she dragged her fingers across the paper, I turned to see Lucy was covered in paint. For a moment I wanted to stop her, make sure she didn't get too messy, restore order. Then I changed my mind.

'Why don't we try using our feet?' I exclaimed, and the children laughed even harder.

I grabbed Lucy and undressed her – leaving her in just a nappy – while Oli pulled off his T-shirt and trousers. The two of them sat in the middle of the paper, plunging hands and feet into the margarine tubs with relish.

'How about you, Han? Do you want another go?'

'Yes please, Mummy.'

I got up and tiptoed towards her across the paper, careful not to smudge the pictures that Oli and Lucy had made. Colours bled into one another, conker brown and sludge green appearing on the paper as the paints pooled together. I could see Lucy heading for the wall and knew there would soon be a messy handprint on it. Paint was already smeared across a coffee table I'd pushed to the side of the room. I'd leave a few marks when I cleaned up later – reminders of memories made on a happy day.

'Can you carry the drip bag for me, please?' I asked Oli as I lifted up Hannah underneath her arms.

He walked towards us and took the bag I'd unhooked. He held onto it tightly, carrying it like a precious relic as I lowered Hannah's feet into the paint.

'It's cold,' she squealed as I lifted her out and we started walking across the paper.

Her feet dangled in the air as I held her. Dipping her down, her feet met the paper as we moved across it together.

'Look, Mummy,' Hannah exclaimed as she turned her head to stare at the pictures she'd left behind.

'What is it?'

'It's like footprints in the sand.'

It was a prayer Hannah knew well. In it, a narrator talks about a dream they've had. Walking across a beach, scenes from their life replay, but as they look back they notice that the two sets of footprints representing God walking beside them dwindle to one at times – particularly during the most difficult periods of the narrator's life. So they ask God why He left when He was needed most, and God replies that He didn't – He was carrying them at their hardest moments when they were too weak to keep on walking.

Hannah smiled up at me as I held her in my arms.

'It is like that, isn't it, Mummy?' she asked again.

'Yes,' I said. 'It's just like that, Han.'

It was a kitchen cupboard that summed up how different our life was now: on one shelf stood packets of cereal, jams and a biscuit barrel, on the other boxes of swabs and syringes, gloves, dressing packs and a sharps box to store used needles. Every time I opened the cupboard door I felt afraid that I would never be able to pick up where I'd left off. I wanted us to have our normal life back, for things to be as they'd been when life was simple and I was sure. But now medicines and equipment jostled for space in my kitchen cupboards with biscuits and baked beans.

Hannah was still too weak to eat or walk and would be for months to come. A wheelchair sat by the front door and a feeding pack was housed in a metal box about a foot long which she was connected to day and night, four hours on, three hours off, via a nasogastric tube. She also needed oxygen constantly and liquid medications every two hours which I gave via her central line or nasogastric tube: captopril for blood pressure, furosemide to combat fluid retention, digoxin to make her heart beat efficiently, ranitidine to stop ulcers forming in her stomach.

Because the central line gave direct access to Hannah's heart, it was vital that it was kept clean. Any kind of infection for a child as weak as her could be fatal and so I had to be scrupulous about 'flushing' the line once a day. This involved cleaning the three smaller lines which ran off the main one coming out of Hannah's chest. Each of the three smaller lines had a cap on the end to which syringes could be attached and it took me up to forty-five minutes to complete the process.

But even with my medical training I could never have prepared myself for those first few weeks at home, and it was the tiny, unanticipated details which threatened to overwhelm me. Just getting Hannah up and down the stairs to bed was difficult because I couldn't carry her as well as a heavy oxygen cylinder. So I'd disconnect her from it before moving her as quickly as possible, knowing she would soon get breathless. After putting her on the sofa or back into bed, I'd run back for the oxygen so that I could reconnect her to it with the minimum of discomfort.

Tiny acts took on a huge significance, like taking off the pieces of tape securing Hannah's nasogastric tube. It had to be done regularly but they chafed her skin and left it so raw that she hated having it done almost as much as I hated having to do it. As Hannah cried, I would try to gently ease the tape away from the raw spots on her cheek, but however careful I was I sometimes couldn't stop her pain.

But it wasn't just Hannah I had to look after now – there were Oli and Lucy to also consider, and once again I'd completely overlooked key details as I'd thought about coming home from the comfort of a hospital ward. For instance something as simple as taking Oli and Lucy into nursery or to the park for a walk was impossible because I couldn't leave Hannah. I was filled with guilt knowing they'd been so excited to have me home and feeling a complete failure now that I was.

Andrew did as much as he could but he'd taken so much time off work while Hannah was in hospital that he couldn't have any more. Mountains of washing up slowly grew and piles of dirty clothes inched upwards. Or I'd open the fridge door and realise we had nearly run out of food before ringing Andrew to give him a hurried list.

'You'll have to leave work ten minutes early so you can stop at the supermarket,' I'd tell him, trying to smooth out the panic in my voice. 'Please don't be late.'

He didn't know that each day I counted down the minutes to 5.30 p.m., almost holding my breath until the moment he walked through the door. When I saw Andrew's face I would feel like crying with relief knowing that he would now look after Oli and Lucy, which meant I just had to focus on Hannah. As I got her ready for bed, he would feed and bath the others before putting them into bed, clearing up the house and cooking us some food.

Even when Oli and Lucy were asleep, though, I hardly saw Andrew. As soon as I'd finally soothed Hannah into sleep I would lie down exhausted on the mattress I used on the floor by her bed, snatching some rest in the hour before preparing her next set of medication. It was hard for both Andrew and me, but we understood that we had to get through the days one by one if we were to hold our family together. In those first few weeks at home, I didn't bath or wash my hair, look in a mirror or iron clean clothes. All I could do was put one foot in front of the other and complete the most crucial tasks.

Days passed and I hardly slept because when I did lie down I felt too agitated to relax. When I finally dropped off I'd soon wake up again to find the house quiet. Feeling my stomach gnaw, I sometimes went to find the food that Andrew had left for me. But as I sat down to try and eat it I'd listen to the silence and feel full of fear that I wouldn't be able to get out of bed again when the alarm next went off.

But even as I began to realise I wasn't coping, I felt too ashamed to admit it. I felt inadequate that I couldn't do everything now when I most needed to. But about two weeks after Hannah came home I finally rang the A&E at Worcester Hospital.

'I need help,' I pleaded down the phone. 'I need someone to come to my house.'

'I'm afraid we can't just send someone out,' a voice said. 'You have to make an appointment before we can assess you.'

'But I can't wait that long. I need help now. Today.'

'I'm sorry but there's really nothing we can do.'

I knew I had to be firm, to make this person listen to me, otherwise I would drown.

'If you don't send someone now then I will bring my daughter to you,' I said as I steadied my voice. 'I cannot cope any more.'

Within an hour my GP, a social worker and two nurses had arrived at my house and arranged for an auxiliary nurse to come to the house for an hour each morning and evening. They couldn't be left alone with Hannah because they weren't trained to look after her central line, but at least I would be able to do some jobs while they were there. It was a start at least, but I still tried to deny what was happening as I got more and more exhausted. It took a few more weeks for things to finally reach rock bottom and for me to realise that unless I changed they would never start back moving up again.

It happened one morning after I'd decided to take Oli and Lucy to the sweet shop. We hadn't been out before and I don't know why I wanted to do it that particular day. Maybe I was desperate to do something normal for them, maybe I wanted to prove that our life could resume the rhythm it had once had – walks in the park, feeding the ducks, nursery and finger painting – a tiny straw to clutch onto as I felt things slip out of my control.

I told the children what we were going to do and Oli started excitedly planning what sweets he wanted. Two hours later we were finally all ready to leave the house and I opened the front door with Hannah and Oli in a buggy and Lucy in a backpack. Hannah's feeding pack was clamped to the pram and there was a small oxygen cylinder in the sling underneath the seat. I also had digoxin, furosemide and codeine with me in case Hannah suddenly deteriorated because I was always ready to phone 999 if she got out of breath or went grey. Hannah's heart condition meant that she could weaken at any time.

Our house was at the end of a cul-de-sac, and almost as soon as we stepped outside we reached a pavement. Easing the pushchair down it, I walked across the road to tip it back up onto the pavement at the other side.

'Ow!' Hannah cried as her feeding line pulled and I heard the oxygen tank bump the pavement.

Breathing deeply, I stopped to check her.

'It's OK, Han,' I soothed. 'We're going to the sweet shop. It won't take long.'

'But I don't want sweets,' she cried. 'I want to go home.'

'No, Mummy!' Oli cried. 'I want to go to the sweet shop.'

I leaned down to Hannah.

'We'll go quickly and then we'll go straight back home. I promise.'

Hannah didn't say anything else as I started walking. I just had to get to the shop, reach it, buy the children some sweets and things would be right again. Step by step, we'd get there.

The minutes dragged by as I walked around two corners and down to the main road. Four side streets to cross – four times down a pavement and four up the other side. Each time, I tried to push the buggy as gently as possible, but Hannah winced with every movement.

'Nearly there,' I kept saying. 'It's not too far now and then we'll go home.'

I wished that a familiar face would appear in front of me as passers-by walked by – someone we knew, anyone who might help. But no one came and I carried on pushing until we reached the top of the hill which led down to the sweet shop. I looked at it below us.

'I'm tired, Mummy,' Hannah wailed. 'I want to go home.'

I stared at the shop. To get there I would have to cross a main road. I could see people going in and out – the door closing and opening, people leaving with bags, mothers with children clutching bright sweet wrappers. I had to get there and prove to us all that we could still function just like the people I could see now. Our world wasn't so different to theirs, surely? Could I just leave the children here and run to the shop? No. Could I ask someone to look after Hannah and take Oli and Lucy? Of course not. The shop was close but it might as well have been on the other side of the Sahara Desert.

'Please, Mummy,' Hannah sobbed. 'Take me home.'

'No!' Oli shouted at her. 'We're going to the shop.'

Their voices snapped into me.

'Please, Mummy,' Hannah shrieked. 'I want to go home.'

I bent down to kiss her, and as I looked at her tear-stained cheek, reality suddenly jolted into me. What was I thinking? Why was I trying to do this? When would I accept that our life had changed? I wasn't going to do any of us any good by trying to paste a carbon copy of our old life over the new. Everything had changed and I must accept it.

I had to give up my expectations and 'rules' about being the perfect mother and wife, giving my children the perfect upbringing. Things had to change and I must discover how best to let that happen. Hannah and I had seen things that had made our world a different place now. Our old life was a skin we had shed and we had to make a new beginning.

As I turned the pram back towards home, I remembered the splashes of paint on the sitting-room coffee table. There were challenges to overcome now, but there were also joys to be tasted more fully. I had to allow myself, Hannah, Oli and Lucy to experience them in our own time.

I pushed Hannah in through the door of the village hall. Inside, mothers and children who'd attended the playgroup I'd run with my friend Karen until Hannah got sick were waiting for us. Although I knew Hannah wouldn't be able to stay long, I wanted her to be here today.

We'd just got back home after ten days in hospital. Hannah had been readmitted after coming down with severe shingles and quickly becoming very poorly. It was potentially very serious for a child like her because any kind of infection makes the heart rate rise. She hated being back in hospital, though – even more when she had to have a catheter inserted through her tummy because livid red shingles had tracked along her groin. I felt desperately sorry that she'd had to return to hospital when she'd only just left. For Hannah, it was a bad place and, however kind the doctors and nurses were, neither they nor I could erase her memories. Going back unsettled her and I only hoped that as she got stronger we could keep our visits to an absolute minimum.

Now I pushed Hannah into the hall and a burst of noise surrounded us as everyone started singing 'Happy Birthday'. I could see a table laid with party plates and hats, balloons dancing above it on strings, presents wrapped in colourful paper and a birthday cake sitting proudly in the middle.

'Who's party is it, Mummy?'

'Yours, Hannah.'

'But it's not my birthday. My birthday isn't until July.'

It was almost three months away but Karen knew that with only three rounds of chemotherapy and such a low heart function, nothing was sure for Hannah. I spoke to Karen on the phone every day and she was the one person I came closest to letting my terror tumble out in front of because while Andrew and I drew strength from each other's constancy we didn't confront our fears together. It was as if speaking them to each other might overwhelm us and so I tried to keep the coiled spring sitting trapped inside me in check as we waited to see if Hannah would stay in remission or there would be an improvement in her heart function.

Each day was a complete unknown and Andrew and I had recently had to travel down to London to meet doctors at Great Ormond Street in case Hannah needed a transplant in the future. They'd told us that she couldn't even be considered for one until she had been in remission from cancer for five years, and cases like hers were so rare that the hospital had only ever performed a handful of transplants in similar circumstances. All that was certain was that keeping the white blood cells low after a transplant to minimise the risk of organ rejection increased the risk of the cancer returning, and if that happened Hannah could not undergo chemotherapy again because a new heart would not be strong enough to cope with it.

So Andrew and I had quietly listened before returning to our life, each of us focused on letting the days and weeks unfold, hoping we might have months and years, knowing nothing was sure. This is what Karen understood and why she had organised today's party.

'I know it's not your birthday, Han,' I said as I pushed her wheelchair towards our waiting friends. 'But everyone wanted to give you an extra one this year because you've been so brave.'

'Does that mean I won't have my real birthday?'

'No. It means you'll have two.'

She grinned as mothers and children surged around us, smiling and cooing words of encouragement as they looked at Hannah.

'Look at your lovely hat!' one mother cried.

'And your beautiful dress,' another said.

They did not need to tell me they understood. They did not need to express in words how sorry they were. All I needed to know was in the faces of these mothers who could easily have shied away from a child who was so unwell – a painful reminder of just how fragile life could be. But these women had not turned away or refused to acknowledge Hannah's illness. No words were needed now because as I looked around me I felt surrounded by love.

On a sunny afternoon in April I took Hannah, Oli and Lucy to our local pub where Andrew was a regular. His friends had decided they wanted to raise money to send Hannah to Disneyland in Paris, and after doing sponsored cycle rides and darts matches some of them were now going to have their heads shaved.

'Will their hair grow back?' Hannah asked as she stared at the huge men whose soft skulls looked as pink as newborns.

'Yes,' I told her.

'When?'

'Soon.'

'Does that mean my hair will grow back too?'

'Yes, Han.'

'When?'

'It will take a little bit longer, but it will, I promise.'

The trip to France was scheduled for June, but just before we were due to leave, Hannah had to go back into hospital again. It was three months since she'd finished her chemotherapy, but after the shingles she'd been in and out with infections – two in her chest and one in her toe. Each had to be taken as seriously as the last and I would leave Andrew to cope with Oli and Lucy because even something as tiny as a gum infection could not go unchecked.

When we finally got home, I was constantly watchful of Hannah – checking her temperature several times a day because it gave me the clearest indication whether her body was fighting an infection or not. If she had to go back into hospital I would stay with her until she was well enough to be discharged and I would continue administering her antibiotics via her central line at home.

By the time we left for Disneyland she was better but still on the antibiotics, so I got onto the the ferry carrying a tin filled with syringes, needles, glass phials of antibiotics and saline packs. When I asked if there was a first aid room we could use, Hannah was delighted to be shown to the captain's cabin where I carefully syringed the drugs into her line as she chatted excitedly about our trip.

We arrived at Disneyland late in the day and put Hannah and Oli into separate beds in the hope that they'd fall asleep quickly. But as we turned off their lamps, the lights in the park suddenly came to life. Outside our windows, Disneyland stretched out into the distance, lights twinkling along the roads, around the houses and at the edges of tramlines.

'Look, Mummy!' Oli cried as he leaped out of bed.

I lifted up Hannah as Andrew grabbed her oxygen cylinder and we walked to the window. I could almost hear her sigh with relief.

'It's Cinderella's castle,' she gasped.

In the days that followed, Hannah decided that what she loved most were the daily parades when her favourite Disney characters came to life. The one she particularly liked was led by furry chipmunks, and each day we'd go to the main square where we'd wait for them to walk up Main Street, leading a procession full of colour and music which ended with huge floats where more characters sat.

But one afternoon, as Hannah watched intently, the chipmunks didn't walk past us. Instead two stopped and held out their huge furry hands as they beckoned her to join the parade. As Hannah tried to stand, I unclipped the lines to her feeding pack even as I wondered how she was ever going to walk. She could still only manage a few steps at home and was so unsteady on her feet that we always used a wheelchair when we went out. But Hannah didn't look back as the two chipmunks took her hands and she got slowly to her feet. Step by tiny step, she walked away from me.

Teetering forwards, Hannah melted into the parade: Mickey Mouse danced, Minnie bobbed her bowed head and smiling furry animals jigged to the music. Hannah looked tiny amid it all but the chipmunks didn't let go of her hands for a moment. They walked at a snail's pace with her as Snow White glided into the square on a huge float, greenery tumbling from its sides and a tiny house perching on the top.

But suddenly the float came to a grinding halt as Snow White got up and started to climb down from it. The procession stretching down Main Street stopped and Hannah watched in wonder as Snow White got off the float, walked across to her and kissed her cheek. A minute later she climbed back on to the float again and it started its journey as the chipmunks helped Hannah walk back to us.

Her eyes were dancing as she sat down in her buggy.

'I was the only child Snow White said hello to, Mummy,' she said in a rush. 'Wasn't she beautiful?'

Snow White didn't know what she'd done that day, just as the mothers at my playgroup couldn't have either. But together they taught me that if you look for love you will find it in many places – sometimes it is steady and enduring and sometimes it is there in a moment you will never forget.

CHAPTER FIVE

Magic in the Air

❀

I think you have to give love as well as get it. You also have to show people so they know you're thinking of them. Sometimes I do that by telling them, but usually it's by giving birthday cards and presents. The people I love are: Mum, who's gentle, Dad, who's strong, Lucy, who's funny, Oli, who's kind, and Phoebe, who's nutty. I also love Grandma and Grandad and Katie my cousin, who's also nutty. I love my family round the world and back again which is very important. You've got to love people whether it's your family or someone else because otherwise you'd have no support and find life very hard.

There's one kind of love that I don't really get, though, and it's the one everyone goes on about – when a girl meets a boy, like *The Prince and Me*. It's a film about a girl who goes to university and falls for a boy who turns out to be a prince. She loves him so much she thinks she'll give up her life to become a princess. But then she realises she's not ready because she wants to study more. So she goes back to being normal and he says he'll wait until she's ready to marry him.

Love Lessons by Jacqueline Wilson is about it too. In it two sisters are home educated until their dad has a stroke and they have to go to school. But they can't get into a good one so they have to go to the lowest of the low and it's hard to start with. Then Prue, the older sister, falls in love with her art teacher Mr Raxberry and they end up kissing. I think that's supposed to be good but I just found it funny that she fancied an old man. The only boy I'd definitely fall in love with would be Zac Efron, but then anybody would fall in love with him. Otherwise I'm not interested. Maybe one day I'll want to fall in love like Cinderella, but not now. There are too many other things to do to worry about that.

At the moment, I'm sitting on my bed in my room and I have to tell you that my bed is a total sticker. I'd never get rid of it. It's four-postered with white wood and pink curtains on the top. I've been told I could have a bed that moves up and down to help when I'm ill because my pillow riser, which lifts me up to help my breathing when it gets bad, can be really uncomfortable then. But there's no way I'm having a different bed.

When we left our last house, I thought I'd never like my new bedroom as much as the one I was leaving because it had more than fifty stickers on the wall. But we had to move because my bedroom was upstairs, which meant I was a bit cut off from everyone whereas now my room is next to the front door so I can hear them coming and going. Mum also got really tired going up and down the stairs all the time to see me in our old house. One day she counted and she'd done it sixty-two times because I was so ill that I could not even turn on the

TV. But my new bedroom was a bit boring when I first moved into it because the walls were dark blue and there was a horrible reddy brown carpet on the floor. I really wasn't looking forward to spending much time in it but then a charity called Make a Wish offered to decorate it for me and asked me to choose paint colours and fabrics. What did I pick? PINK, of course!

I forgot all about my room when I went to Acorns. I go there at the end of every month and the longest I've stayed was two weeks, although it's usually four nights. The nurses and carers there are really nice and first came to see me when I was in hospital after my heart got bad. They don't accept every child who goes into hospital and so they had to do tests and have meetings before accepting me. But I'm glad they did because I really enjoy it at Acorns. I can rest and Mum and Dad have one too, which is important because they're tied to me at home and so while I'm away they get to do what they want.

Acorns is a hospice and a lot of the children who go there are in wheelchairs or on food pumps. Most of them are little although there are some older kids who bash the walls with their wheelchairs when they race up and down the corridors. Some children die there, and one was a baby girl who I liked very much. She was very cute with wild hair and I missed her when she died. I also thought a lot about her mum and dad, who were really nice, and the great big loss that they must have felt when she had gone.

It made me feel sad but Acorns isn't usually like that and I laugh all the time there – especially with Paul who does night shifts and is a nutter. There's also lots of things to do like go in the pool, which is so warm you can never get cold. In the summer we have a sports day – just a bit easier – and water fights. There are also Playstations, Sing Stars and an art room. But the best thing is the food which you can smell cooking because the kitchen is right next to the sitting room and the door is always open. Martin, Sally, Corby and Jane are the cooks and they're really nice because although you're not allowed in the kitchen when they're making lunch you can ask to cook things when they're not busy. I once made a chocolate cake. The best thing, though, is that you can ask for something else if you don't like what's been made and have whatever you want – even pizza.

When I first went to Acorns, Mum went with me for weekend stays. But then I decided I wanted to go for longer and Mum wasn't sure she could come because there was Oli, Lucy, Phoebe, Dad, the horses, chickens, Ted and Tails McFluff to look after as well as me. At first I was a bit worried about going on my own but then I realised it would be a breeze because Acorns is like being at home. There are TVs, big comfy sofas and always someone to talk to. They really listen to what you say and I've even helped do things like pick new duvet covers for the rooms. I also suggested they got some lava lamps for our bedrooms because they wanted something a bit more sensory and although there's a lot of stuff they can't have because of safety restrictions I thought those would be OK. I like having a light on in my room at night if I'm not well so I thought other kids might too.

The only thing I don't like about Acorns sometimes is that no one else my age seems to go there so I play with a girl who's ten, which is quite a lot younger. She's really nice but sometimes I wish there was another thirteen-year-old to muck around with. If I feel like that, though, I have a chat with Yasmin, who's my link carer and really nice, or one of the two Clares or one of the two Helens, or Andrea or Sharnie, and I feel all right again.

Anyway, I was having so much fun at Acorns that I'd forgotten all about my room by the time Mum, Oli, Lucy and Phoebe came to pick me up. But when they walked in to see me, Phoebe shouted that they had come in a big white car.

Mum's car is blue so I wondered what she was on about.

'And the man driving it has a big hat,' she yelled.

Then I knew something was up so I went to the front door and what did I see? A massive white stretch limo, that's what!

'What's this for?' I asked Mum.

'Well, you've always wanted to ride in one so today's the day,' she told me and I couldn't believe it.

We piled into the car where there were disco lights flashing and music playing which was brilliant until Oli felt sick halfway home and we had to stop. I didn't feel too bad for him, though, because he'd drunk nearly all the Coke on the way up to Acorns so it was his own fault.

But I still didn't realise what was happening when we got home and I walked into the house. Then I opened the door to my room and saw what Make a Wish had done. The whole room had been decorated – pink walls, pink carpet, pink curtains. It was so amazing I didn't dare to touch anything. That was a year ago and I'm still really pleased that Make a Wish did my room.

I think that day is one of my best memories, and another is meeting Prince Charles after I got picked to go with some other children to Clarence House. I was expecting his house to be massive but it was smaller than I thought it would be. Still, though, I was going to meet a prince so I'd put on my smartest clothes – a long purple skirt with flowers on it and a white top with fake fur around the wrists. As everyone waited for him, I kept thinking there would be some trumpets or something to let us know he'd arrived. Instead I turned around and there he was.

Mum was with me and we'd bought a present to give the Prince. I felt really nervous as I handed over what we'd brought – biscuits, jam and some kind of alcohol. (I wouldn't want to be given alcohol because I had a sip of sherry once and it gave me a headache but Mum thought Prince Charles would like it.)

'Is this good?' he asked as he looked at the bottle.

I didn't know what to say because I hadn't tasted it so I told him Mum liked it and he laughed. Then he carried on chatting to me and I was really surprised because I thought he'd be really strict and not say much. But he was very nice and looked really smart in his uniform with buttons, a chain and coloured stripes on it. He was wearing it because he'd been doing investitures before he met all the children and the only thing that really surprised me about Prince Charles was that he was much shorter than I thought he'd be. In fact he was only a bit taller than Mum and his hands were really big with fingers as fat as sausages.

But maybe my best memory is of the Christmas just gone because it was so great. The year before, I'd only had my pacemaker in for six months and was still so ill that I couldn't eat anything except a couple of carrots. I wanted to have more, but when the food got close to my mouth, I couldn't eat it I knew I couldn't just sit there and watch everyone else so Mum carried me to the lounge to wait until they had finished and came to sit down with me.

It was so horrible because Christmas lunch is my favourite but I just couldn't get the food into my mouth. Have you ever had that? It's like a little voice is whispering as you push the fork towards you, saying, 'Don't do it.' That's why last Christmas was so great because I was much better by then and had absolutely everything: turkey with all the trimmings, stuffing, gravy, vegetables and sausages wrapped in bacon. Afterwards we had a Christmas pudding which Dad covered in whisky and set alight. Blue flames flickered around it, which was excellent.

Mum told me to wait a bit before I had some, which she does because she knows I'll get stomach pains if I eat too much. (That's what Dad forgot when he gave me his wonder stew.) So I waited, and when I finally had the pudding it tasted so good that I'll never forget it. It just shows what you can do when you really want to.

꩜

Our new life got better the longer we lived it together, and by the time Hannah turned five in the July after we got home from hospital she and I had developed a routine about her medications and care. Each tiny step forward felt huge and my confidence slowly grew as I learned to flush the central line more quickly. Hannah hadn't had a single infection in it, which was unusual, and I knew I had to trust that I was doing it well – just as I had to listen to the instinct that was telling me more and more strongly that I could not constantly watch over her.

Early on, I realised that Hannah's illness could make or break our family. Just as many marriages crack under the strain, so do the childhoods of many siblings of sick children as parents pour everything into them and leave little for the rest. Of course there were days when Hannah was particularly ill at home or back in hospital, having lost weight or needing a feeding tube replacement, when my focus was solely on her. But I also knew Oli and Lucy had just as much right to happiness and security as Hannah and I must save some of my energy for them.

I understood the parents I'd seen in hospital who took their children halfway across the world in the search for a cure but knew I would never be one of them. I respected those parents' choice and would do everything I could to care for Hannah, fight for her treatment and make decisions in her best interests. But I also knew that the right thing for my family was to give Hannah, Oli and Lucy as normal a life as possible – one that included and made allowances for Hannah's illness, but also gave space for her brother and sister to be carefree children. Their lives were healthy, and like all children they were rushing through them. I had to allow them to do that. The future was uncertain but the best thing for all of us was to live our life believing that Hannah would one day be well again, otherwise nothing would make sense.

Bit by bit I started spending time with Oli and Lucy in the two hours when Hannah was off her feeding pack during the afternoon. At first it was just a few minutes, but it gradually built up to about half an hour. After putting Hannah in front of a favourite television programme, I'd go up to Oli's room. I knew my full attention was worth a whole day of treats to him and so we'd take crisps, cheese and apples up to his room before tucking sheets around the bottom of his bed on stilts to make Lucy a fairy castle to play in. Then Oli and I would build towers of Lego or he would whizz up and down the ladder to his bed as I watched.

We also started making short trips to the park where I would play with Oli and Lucy as Hannah sat in her buggy. I wanted her to carry on learning the lessons that any other child her own age would, and patience was one of them. Just as a mother knows her baby's cry, I was always alert, ready to drop everything if Hannah needed me urgently, but I made myself stop responding to every call. The need to constantly comfort her could become almost overwhelming if I wasn't careful and I knew it would not help her, Oli or Lucy to cosset her in my constant attention.

Now we were home, Hannah and I had an ongoing conversation about her illness, and while she never complained about it I knew she didn't always like watching her brother and sisters venture out bit by bit into the world.

'Am I still poorly, Mummy?' she'd ask as we sat at the kitchen table drawing. 'Why isn't anyone else poorly too?'

'Well, the bugs in your blood made you ill, Han,' I'd reply. 'That's why you have to take all your pills because they'll help to get you better.'

'Will I go to school soon?'

'We hope so. Your heart is still poorly but we hope it's going to get better.'

Hannah stopped what she was doing and looked at me.

'You know that if I go to heaven I will be with grandma and grandpa until you come and there will be lots of sweeties, animals and trees?'

'Yes, my darling.'

However often we had the conversation, I would always try to still myself inside when we spoke – knowing I must be honest and open with Hannah but railing against the fact that

I had to be. It made me inexpressibly sad to hear her talk in such a way but Hannah was as quietly accepting as she always had been. She knew she couldn't go outside for too long in the cold or run around with Oli and Lucy because she had to live a different kind of life. But although she could easily have thrown a tantrum or sulked, screamed or shouted about it, she never did.

There were moments, though, when her vulnerabilities shone through, as did mine because although I'd tried to lock away the fear and worry inside me, my feelings had to come out somewhere. That is why my teeth had got worse and worse after Hannah left hospital and eventually they were so bad that I had all my top ones removed because the dentist couldn't save them. I was thirty-four, had dentures and all I could feel was relief that I was no longer in pain.

But although I didn't stop to let myself think about it, there were days when I couldn't contain myself, and one came when I felt so exhausted that I started crying in front of the children. I don't know why it happened and I'd never done it before. But I can clearly remember sitting at the top of the stairs with the three children around me.

'Mummy's very tired,' I sobbed. 'And I want you to go to bed now.'

Their eyes were wide as they looked quizzically at my tears. They knew it was far too early for them to go to bed. The sun was still shining. We had not eaten tea or had a bath yet. This was not how things usually were.

'It's all right, Mummy,' Hannah said. 'I'll help you.'

She was wearing her oxygen line as usual, attached by a long thin tube to the converter in her room which had replaced the cylinders she had come home from hospital with. The converter was a box that looked a bit like a small washing machine which sucked oxygen out of the air and delivered it to Hannah through a tube under her nose. She wore it constantly because her heart wasn't strong enough to properly oxygenate her blood.

But now Hannah slipped off the oxygen line as she took Oli's hand and fright pulsed through me.

'I'm going to put you into bed while Mummy puts Lucy in hers,' she said softly to her brother, and I watched her for a moment – torn between telling her to put the line back on and knowing she couldn't be cooped up in the confines of her illness every minute of every day.

I had to let her be.

As Hannah walked slowly away with her brother, I wiped my face and took Lucy into her room where I settled her before walking back to Oli's. He was lying on his raised bed and Hannah, who couldn't make the climb, was sitting at the bottom in a plastic chair. A book was open in her hands and Oli was leaning out of the side of the bed to look at the pictures as she read to him – the words coming out in breathy chunks.

'We've got halfway through,' she said softly as I stood at the door.

I went back into the hallway to pick up Hannah's oxygen line before going back into Oli's room and putting it on her again. She breathed deeply as the oxygen hissed softly through the line.

'Why don't I help you finish the story?' I said as I sat down beside her.

I pressed my face to the glass panel in the top of the door as it closed. Six months after leaving hospital, Hannah was on the other side being led into a classroom by a teacher for her first day back at school. I'd registered her at a tiny primary in a village called Whitbourne, about ten miles from Worcester where we were looking for a house to buy.

It was a small village with a school surrounded by stone walls, a village hall sitting on a green, a pub, river, shop and a scattering of houses. I wanted my children to walk to school, run barefoot on grass, eat boiled eggs for breakfast from chickens which roamed in the garden. It was a dream I'd always had, but Hannah had taught me that we couldn't put it off for another week, month or year. Andrew and I were going to create the life we wanted for our children today instead of waiting for a tomorrow that might never come.

So while I house hunted, Hannah was going to go to school for a few hours on as many mornings as she could manage. Before she started, I'd explained to the staff that Hannah's heart condition meant she might suddenly go pale or feel faint.

So for the first few weeks, at least, I was going to attend school with her, and although we'd been 'practising' for school so she could be off her oxygen for a few hours, a cylinder would be stored in her classroom just in case she needed it.

I stared at her through the window – still very skinny, Hannah was dwarfed by the backpack she was carrying which contained her feed. Her nasogastric tube was stuck to the side of her cheek and she wore a bobble hat to keep her head warm. I wanted to cheer as I watched her sit down at a table with two other children.

A couple of hours later I arrived back at the class to take her outside for break time. At the start of the day I'd pushed Hannah to the school steps in her wheelchair, but now she wanted to walk. We edged our way twenty feet into the playground and sat down on a bench near the door as children peered shyly before getting braver and walking up to talk to Hannah.

'What's that?' a little boy asked, as he pointed to her feeding tube.

'It's my food. I can't eat enough.'

'Where does it go?'

'Into my tummy.'

'Can we look at your backpack?'

'Yes,' said Hannah matter-of-factly.

'What's that?' another child asked, pointing to the wiggly bag which hung around her neck holding the tubes from her central line.

'It's for my medicine,' Hannah told them seriously.

'Why do you need that?'

'Because I have a poorly heart.'

'Where's your hair?' a little girl asked.

'It fell off,' said Hannah.

'Oh.'

Soon all the questions had been asked and Hannah became just another classmate. My heart leapt with joy.

~

Hannah pressed her face to the window of the plane.

'Where's Father Christmas?' she said. 'I can't see him.'

We were coming in to land on a trip to Scotland with a group from Birmingham Children's Hospital. Today felt very special. Hannah's fifth birthday had been spent in hospital so this was our first chance to celebrate something as a family, and she, Oli and Lucy could barely contain themselves – especially after meeting a very special person on the way up to RAF Kinloss.

'This is Captain Christmas!' a voice had boomed out of the cabin speakers soon after we'd boarded and a ripple of excitement had rushed through the expectant children.

'I'm going to need your help to get off the ground because Santa Claus is waiting! So I want everyone to make a big noise to get the plane into the air.'

Children cheered as we soared into the sky, and soon Oli, Lucy, Hannah, Andrew and I were invited to go and meet Captain Christmas. We walked into the cockpit to find him waiting – snow on the dashboard, lights twinkling and an elf sitting in the next seat.

'He might look like Father Christmas but he's not,' the elf said as he gestured at Captain Christmas's red coat and white beard. 'He's his brother and he's taking you to see Father Christmas because he knows that some of you might not be in your own beds on Christmas Eve.'

Wide-eyed and even more excited, the children had gone back to their seats, and now Hannah watched as we came in to land. On the runway below she could see dozens of figures in fancy dress standing in a line.

'Where is he?' she cried again.

'He'll be here soon,' I told her. 'Captain Christmas will make sure of it.'

After the plane had come to rest, Oli, Lucy and other well siblings walked down the steps to be greeted by the volunteers in costume who were going to look after them for the day. Then Hannah and other sick children were taken off the plane in an armchair lift before being driven to a huge hall.

Inside they found tables laden with food, 'snow' on the ground and streamers tumbling from the ceiling. The children gasped in delight as Andrew, me and the other parents were ushered to seats and told we didn't have to do a thing for the rest of the afternoon because doctors and nurses from Birmingham were on hand. Quiet astonishment filled all our faces as brothers and sisters dug into huge bowls of sweets and crisps, while sick children were given small morsels of food which had been specially prepared for their tiny appetites. If, like Hannah, they couldn't eat, the volunteers helped them colour in pictures or 'dance' to the disco music that was playing. Laughter and shouts filled the air, and within an hour the whole hall was strewn with debris as the children clustered around a huge English Shepherd which had tinsel in his tail and was giving them rides.

'The reindeers are coming …' a voice boomed out, and children rushed to the windows.

Far in the distance, at the other side of the airfield, were six reindeers pulling Father Christmas in a sledge.

'He's coming to see us,' children cried in excitement as the sledge drew closer and closer before Father Christmas finally strode into the hall.

'Happy Christmas, children,' he cried. 'Did my brother bring you here?'

Hannah looked completely overwhelmed, Oli and Lucy wiggled with delight and I remembered last year when Hannah had been too weak to even sit up when Father Christmas came to see her. Now she held on to the 'mouse' and 'fairy' looking after her as he came inside and children rushed at him.

'Now you need to come up to see me one by one,' he said with a laugh as he sat down on a throne. 'Because although I don't normally give out presents before Christmas Day, I think you've been all good enough to have one early.'

Each child was given a present before some of the well ones were put into a fire engine, water cannons firing as they drove around the airfield, while others patted the reindeers. It was too cold for Hannah to go outside but she sat and watched the others until dusk finally began to fall and a voice shouted that Father Christmas had to leave.

'He needs some help getting off the ground,' the children were told, and they started cheering.

The lights of the sleigh shone as Father Christmas galloped across the airfield into the distance, gradually dimming as he rode further and further into the darkness before suddenly disappearing. Seconds later the lights rose into the air and the children stared in wonder as Father Christmas 'flew' into the night sky.

Now it was time to get back on the plane as Captain Christmas appeared in his flight helmet to welcome us all back on board.

'Now don't forget to say goodbye,' he told the cabin.

We looked out of the windows. In the darkness the fancy dress figures had lined up once again on the runway, each wearing a glove with tiny lights embedded in it which twinkled as we rose into the air – scores of hands waving us goodbye, ordinary people who had given their time to wish us a Happy Christmas.

CHAPTER SIX

Live the Life You Love

The news is full of stories about MPs' expenses and it's got me thinking about what I'd do if I was Prime Minister. The first thing would be to sack all the MPs who have got us into debt and fiddled their expenses. But these are the others:

- Make the government pay for children's hospice care like Acorns because they don't and I think that's really bad.
- Get more people into work because there are less jobs now during the credit crisis and the government should be helping people get theirs back.
- Give everyone a free holiday worth up to £1,000. Some people can't afford a holiday and everyone is stressed right now.
- Stop charging for parking at hospital because it's really expensive. No one should pay because if they're at a hospital they're either going to work there or visiting someone who's ill.
- Stop hospital parking attendants being so fussy. The taxi which takes me to hospital school can hardly stop to let me out before the driver gets in trouble.

- Give every child a year's supply of chocolate.
- Give children good homes. I see children at Acorns who can't move or talk but they've got good mums and dads and that's a lot compared to some who are living in homes with parents who don't love them.

I thought that last one up after going to visit the British Heart Foundation to meet other kids like me. I thought it was going to be really boring and we'd all have to sit around telling each other what was wrong with us. But instead we did activities and just chatted when we felt like it, which was good. I met one girl about my age who'd had a heart transplant and told me she'd just had to go back into hospital because her body was trying to reject her heart, which made me feel a bit funny. Mostly, though, I liked meeting other kids who were all as different as me. It reminded me that I'm not the only one with a bad heart, and the world opened up a bit – I didn't feel so closed in. It was also good because we talked about the here and now, not the future, and that's what I like to do – take every day as it comes, which means you mostly enjoy them instead of worrying.

Sometimes of course I think about the transplant again but it's usually only when I've been feeling really ill, like after I went to the horse show with Lucy. I had not been that ill for a long time and it took ages to feel better. I'm still a bit tired but I'm back to being me, and even though I've been told I'll get sicker if I don't have the operation and my illness might go away if I do I still know that I'm not having it. When people keep asking why I said no, I wonder if they really understand what it's like to be ill when you're a child because if they did then I don't think they'd go on about my decision so much.

My earliest memory is of going to Disneyland when I was nearly five – the train, the big castle and all the people walking below us looking like one of those photos in Harry Potter where the pictures have moving people in them. After that I can remember being at home and doing my school work while Mum was in the kitchen. I used to sit at a desk underneath a window and could hear noise from outside. But other than that a lot of my memories are about hospitals: going for check-ups, having blood tests, Mum taking the tape off my nasogastric tube when I was little, which hurt so much that I screamed, the Vitamin K injections I had to have in my leg after my heart got worse, which really hurt, that kind of thing.

I also remember having to go to hospital all the time for check-ups, which I didn't like. The doctors were always nice but being in hospital is boring so imagine what it feels like if you have to go there all your life. I remember one doctor who looked like Chris Tarrant off *Who Wants to Be a Millionaire?* I think he might have dyed his hair because a friend of my mum's did that and you could see all the grey when she hadn't done it. I've dyed my hair before and wondered if I'd get told off when I went to school with it. No one seemed to notice except one of the teachers who gave me a slightly funny look. I wondered what I'd say if she asked about it so I decided to tell her it was permanent and I couldn't wash it out. In fact, I want to do my hair again now but can't decide whether to go chestnut or blonde.

Anyway, what I mean about the transplant is that when you've been ill you learn to think about things because you have so much time to. I know that if my heart gets worse I will probably get more and more tired, short of breath and go to bed. That's what happens when your heart gives up. But I'm not going to collapse on the floor without a fight and I don't think about it all the time because if I did I wouldn't do anything, would I? I don't go around thinking, 'Oh my gosh, I might die this week,' because there would be no point in living otherwise and that's what I want to do. I made my decision to suit me and I knew Mum and Dad were happy with it. They would have gone with whatever I wanted, and that was to be back at home. I did not want another operation or to have to stay in hospital for ages. It was weird, though, when I was finally allowed to come home and Mum came in to say goodnight when I was in my own bed for the first time in ages.

'It's nice to be home, isn't it?' she asked.

To be honest, I felt strange because I'd wanted to be back so much and now I didn't know what to do with myself. It's like you have to learn to be at home again when you've been away a long time. But I was happy that Mum was happy and I was too because the whole hospital thing was over. It just took a bit of getting used to being at home, but even then I couldn't get away from being ill because I had to take meds all the time. It's a big thing for me, and at the moment I take seven pills in the morning, two at lunchtime and five in the evening. It's not that much compared to what I've taken before – sometimes more than thirty pills a day at 8 a.m., 10 a.m., 12 p.m., 2 p.m., 4 p.m., 6 p.m. and 8 p.m.

It might not sound a lot, but believe me, if you have to do it every day then it gets to be a real pain. I know I have to take the meds because they're my crutches and I'd fall if I didn't have them. But sometimes I just wish I could be free because the meds remind me I'm ill and it's one of the things that puts me off having a transplant because I'd have to take anti-rejection drugs for the rest of my life. I hate taking pills and occasionally it annoys me so much that I've refused to take them. Mum doesn't force me because she understands that I've made my mind up, but I know she wants me to take them.

Don't get me wrong, it's sad if people waste their life by feeling sorry for themselves when they're ill, and I hope I'm not like that. All I'm saying is that being in hospital for a short while is OK and there's a lot to play with if you're a young child, but it gets harder as you get older. You see the same walls every day and know what's going to happen. The worst thing, though, about being ill when you are older is that you know what you're missing.

I'm lucky because at least I got better after having leukaemia and went backwards and forwards to hospital until I was at the back of the queue for a while. Then my heart got worse, but even then there were good things like going to Acorns and having a new bedroom. They might sound small to someone who hasn't been ill but they're big and you have to be grateful for what you've got because even if it's not a lot there's always someone worse off than you. Think of the children lying in hospital now who are going to die. So don't get me wrong when I say it's bad being ill because I'm not the worst off and I don't feel sad about it all the time. But I suppose what I'm really saying is that sometimes I get bored of it.

A rush of nerves filled me as I stared at the paper I'd just signed. It was a letter telling Hannah's headmaster that I was taking her out of school because I was going to educate her at home. It was a huge decision and I suddenly wondered if I was doing the right thing.

We'd moved to Whitbourne days before Christmas 2000 into one of four semi-detached houses which stood in a line on a hill overlooking fields. The house needed some work but the view was beautiful and the big garden was perfect for the children. We'd arrived to find the electricity had been cut off but I knew we were home as I lit some candles.

In the months that followed, Oli and Lucy had been registered at the nursery attached to the village school and Hannah had continued to go as often as she could. She'd also come off permanent oxygen and got a little stronger. But as much as I wanted her to be well enough for school, she became increasingly tired and anxious about her limits.

'Will I feel too sick in class today, Mummy?' she'd ask. 'Will someone knock me over? I don't want to fall down.'

After months spent with other sick children, returning to school had made Hannah acutely aware of how difficult she found it to keep up. She knew she was being left behind and it didn't surprise me that she sometimes got angry as she watched Oli and Lucy begin to explore the world around us. Soon after moving to Whitbourne we'd bought a pony because I'd ridden as a child and wanted Oli and Lucy to learn. To keep the cost down, I'd bought a former riding school pony and agreed to muck out a friend's horse in return for a place for ours in her field. Learning to ride, though, was just one of the new things that Oli and Lucy were doing. They were also beginning to ride scooters and bikes, skip, hop and jump on the trampoline in the garden. Hannah had to be put on it and bounced gently, and although she was beginning to walk more she still couldn't go far.

But it was only after her calm nature erupted into a terrible rage that I knew I had to do something. It happened one morning as Hannah stood in a doorway beside Lucy while I did up their shoes before school. I don't know what provoked Hannah but suddenly she lashed out and I looked up to see Lucy's head smash into the door frame. Springing forward, I reached up to push Hannah away from her sister and she stumbled, crashing into the other side of the door. Blood spurted from a cut on Lucy's head as I turned to Hannah, and red hot anger filled me.

'What are you doing?' I shouted. 'Why did you hurt your sister?'

She didn't say a word as I yelled and felt my hands shaking with rage. But my anger died away as I took Lucy to the bathroom to butterfly stitch her cut. I'd almost lost control and couldn't allow it to happen again.

'Mummy knows she was wrong to grab you and I promise never to do it again,' I said to Hannah later. 'But you must also promise me that you will never hit Lucy like that.'

'I won't,' she said.

'Why did you do it, Han?'

'I don't know,' she said, as if bewildered by my question.

Hannah's calm acceptance of her illness was being pushed to its limits and I knew I had to stop trying to fit her life into a box that it didn't suit. As much as I wanted her to be at school, it was obvious that it was too much and Hannah herself was trying to tell me what she wanted so why couldn't I listen to her?

It was then that I'd heard about home schooling and the parents who educated their children themselves. I'd always thought school was compulsory but now learned that, while parents had a legal duty to ensure their children are educated, it could be done at school or home. A small but growing number of parents across the UK were choosing to home educate their children and I wondered if this was what Hannah needed.

But could I really do something which went against all the 'rules' I'd been taught? Take a step so far out of the mainstream? Before Hannah had got ill I'd lived my life like everyone else – caring for my children, working, paying bills – and

I'd liked it that way. I wasn't sure if I was brave enough to make such a big decision for both Hannah and me. For her, it meant being cut off from classmates, but I knew I could make sure we stayed in touch with the school and met other parents with children who were home educated. For me, it was a big commitment because once I started teaching Hannah I wouldn't be able to return to work for as long as she was with me and it wouldn't be just her physical recuperation that I would be responsible for.

But although Andrew thought the idea was too way out at first and I knew other people would feel the same, the more I thought about it, the more sure I felt. At home, Hannah could learn at her own pace and gain her strength rather than having her confidence knocked by not keeping up at school. She faced challenges many other children didn't and I had to trust my judgement that this decision was right for her. It would be the last part of the jigsaw, and however strange other people might find it to keep Hannah at home with me, I knew what was right for her. When I explained how I felt, Andrew had agreed and I took a deep breath now as I picked up the letter and slipped it into an envelope. I would take it with me to school when I took Hannah in to pick up Oli and Lucy.

Walking to the front door, a feeling of liberation filled me as I wrapped my fingers around the envelope. This was another lesson that Hannah was going to help me learn and now we were going to live the life we loved, however different it might be to the one we had had before. This was the right choice for Hannah and that was all that counted.

'Are you ready?' I called to her as I opened the front door.

The envelope was safe in my pocket. Soon we would start on the next stage of our journey together.

While the future was still uncertain, home schooling made me think very deeply about it. Hannah continued to have regular blood tests to check she was still in remission and heart scans to monitor her progress. But although there were no guarantees, I knew she was getting stronger as I asked myself what I wanted Hannah to learn for the future.

To me, education meant not just sitting with a pen and paper, so as Hannah's sixth birthday approached I started teaching her how to look after the chickens and put plates in the dishwasher. I also tried to make lessons come alive as much as possible, so if we were doing history I would take her to see the Hereford Mappa Mundi – a medieval map of the world that we stared at together in the city's cathedral. To help with maths I gave her coins to count or asked her to double the quantity of flour we were using in a recipe to make the numbers into something real for her.

Food was also a big part of our learning because it remained a problem for Hannah, and I tried to re-engage her interest in it as I taught her. Months after coming out of hospital, she would only eat 'easy' foods like yoghurt and ice cream and still needed the feeding pack. But Hannah had to learn how to eat again because children can become almost phobic about food after going so long without it during chemotherapy. Eating also required a lot of energy for someone with a weak heart like Hannah's, so I had to find ways to make it easier for her.

To help with chewing and swallowing, I started mincing her food into purees before putting them on a plate – a tiny brown pile of pureed mince, another of orange carrot and another of green peas. That way she could see the 'meal' she was trying to eat, and slowly but surely Hannah started to eat a little more. Soon her strength had improved, and within months of starting home schooling she was able to walk outside instead of using her wheelchair and had also come off the feeding pack during the day. She would still need it at night for about another year as she progressed through eating small chunks to whole food, and Hannah would be about nine before I could take her for her first pizza.

But in the meantime I sparked her interest in food by making vegetable growing a big part of our home tuition. Hannah watched as I cut turf in the garden to create a vegetable plot before helping me to plant potatoes, peas, broccoli, carrots, cabbage and cauliflower. In the greenhouse we grew tomatoes, cucumbers, peppers, squash and spaghetti fruits – which looked like a pumpkin until they were cut open to reveal long strands of flesh which Oli and Lucy ate from a

single plate, giggling as they met in the middle of a single
strand like *Lady and the Tramp*.

We also picked plums and apples from trees in our
garden, fed the chickens every day and Hannah helped to
water the plants. After moving to Whitbourne we'd also had
an extension built which housed a big kitchen overlooking
the garden. In it was a pine table, blue and white checked
curtains and an Aga as well as a sofa where Hannah rested
during the day. She still needed a lot of sleep and sometimes
when I put Lucy down for a rest on a soft blue mesh swing
seat in the afternoon I'd put Hannah in with her. Pegging
sheets around it to protect them from the sun, I'd swing them
both to sleep.

When they woke up they'd potter around the garden
together and I'd watch them through the French windows in
the kitchen. Standing by the vegetable plot, they'd throw
scraps to keep the chickens away before reaching up to snaf-
fle peas in their pods. Then the two of them would teeter
across the lawn to the water butt where they'd dip the peas for
a quick wash before popping the whole pod into their mouths.

Hannah seemed to enjoy being at home with me, so much
so that friends called her my little shadow because wherever
I was she was close by, and it made me glad to see her
flourish even though there were times when I wondered if
she was enjoying it a little too much. It usually happened
when I took her down to the village school for break times
and listened to her delightedly tell the other children that
they could have lessons at home too if they wanted.

'You don't have to go to school,' she'd say to her friends, who stared at her in amazement.

On the way back home I'd try to think of ways to convince her to stop her being so enthusiastic as I wondered what the other mothers were going to say when their children decided they weren't going back to school either.

But I was pleased that Hannah seemed to thrive on being at home with me and our unusual lessons. Perhaps her favourite was to watch me digging potatoes and she knew there was one enemy in particular who might spoil her fun – slugs. So at night we'd go outside in our dressing gowns and wellies, holding a paraffin lamp to light up the ground and kitchen tongs to pick up the slugs.

'If we throw them over the hedge they'll come back again tomorrow, won't they?' Hannah would ask, just to make sure that we really had to consign the slugs to their demise in a jar of beer that I was carrying.

'Yes, Han,' I'd tell her.

'OK, Mummy,' she'd say and I'd hear a plop as the slug hit the beer.

When we'd searched for all the slugs we could find, Hannah would finally go inside, safe in the knowledge that her potatoes were protected for another day.

Today was a day that Hannah had spent two years longing for. In the months after her central line had been put in when she first fell ill, it had been in almost constant use. But as time had passed, Hannah had grown stronger and learned to take her heart medications in tablet form so it was needed less. Her heart function had also improved a little, and when the line finally went unused for three months her doctors had decided it could be removed.

We'd gone into hospital to have it done just before her seventh birthday but because the central line had been in place for so long, it had embedded into the skin on Hannah's chest and we'd had to stay in for the site to be monitored after the line was removed. The procedure also involved a general anaesthetic – something Hannah hadn't had since her heart was damaged and extremely risky for her. But she was anaesthetised with a cardiac team on stand-by and the operation was a success.

Hannah had hated being in hospital for her birthday but having the line removed was important because she had never been able to get it wet, which had stopped her from doing so many things she wanted to. For two long years she hadn't had a splashy bath or gone swimming, run through the sprinkler in the garden or played in the paddling pool. Removing it also meant she was finally free of the line coming out of her chest and the 'wiggly' bag holding the connecting tubes which had constantly hung around her neck.

Strange as it sounds, part of me almost dreaded the removal of the line even though I was happy for Hannah. For so long it had been there if she got an infection or her heart worsened – an instant entry point into her body for Hannah to receive rapid and powerful treatment, a safety net that had always been there to catch her. Now I knew it was time to move on from the red alert mode I'd been in for so long – constantly watchful, always ready to drop everything if she got worse, on the look-out for any signs of a recurrence of her leukaemia or worsening of her heart – to amber, from a state of high anxiety to a place where I could almost dare to hope the crisis had passed. I wondered how I'd learn to ease myself out of the constant adrenalin rush I was used to even as I knew that Hannah was moving into a new stage of her recovery, which meant I must too because our life was moving on in more ways than one. Andrew had got a new job which would take him away from home a lot during the week and I would be alone with the children. It was a new phase for all of us.

Now, after several days at home during which Hannah had constantly examined the incision site to check it was healing, her scab was finally starting to transform into a pink scar and it was time for her to have what she'd been longing for – a bubble bath.

'Can Oli come in with me?' she'd asked me that morning.

'Of course.'

'And will you let us shut the door?'

'Maybe. But you must promise not to stand up in the bath.'

'I won't.'

Hannah looked seriously at me for a moment.

'Do you mind if we make a mess?'

'No.'

'What if it's a really big one?'

'That's OK. Just try not to flood the kitchen, Han.'

'OK, Mummy.'

Hannah was beside herself as I ran the bath and filled it to the brim with bubbles – so high that neither she nor Oli would be able to make a bubble beard because they were already up to their chins. After standing Oli in the bath, I sat Hannah down because she was still so wobbly on her feet.

'Will you shout for me if anyone slips?' I asked Oli. 'If you promise to do that then I'll shut the bathroom door.'

'Yes, Mummy,' he yelled in excitement.

I wondered what on earth I was doing leaving a five-and-a-half-year-old and his seven-year-old sister in a bath full of bubbles equipped with everything from water colourings to fizzing soaps. But I couldn't stop myself from smiling as I went downstairs and heard peals of laughter and howls of hysteria start to pour through the kitchen ceiling. It sounded like pure joy crystallised in a sound, and as I watched water begin to stain the kitchen ceiling I knew I didn't care if it came down. Oli and Hannah's joy was like a bright light rushing through me.

'Can you get me out of the bath please, Mummy?' Hannah shouted about half an hour later. 'Oli's done it but I can't.'

I walked up the stairs and braced myself for what I was going to find. Opening the door, I looked ahead and saw Hannah's eyes looking at me from just above the edge of the bath. There were bubbles everywhere, streaks of brightly coloured soap up the wall and water all over the floor. Oli had disappeared, leaving his big sister to face the music, and Hannah's eyes were anxious as she peered at me, her hair sitting up in tufts on her head.

'I'm sorry, Mummy,' she said.

I looked at her and smiled.

'It's OK, Han,' I said as I went to lift her out of the bath. 'We made a deal, didn't we?'

'Really?'

'Yes! I said you could have a big bath and you've had it.'

I wrapped her in a towel and lifted her up.

'Did you have fun?'

'It was great,' she said, her eyes shining. 'Can we do it again?'

I smiled as we passed the door to Oli's bedroom and she leaned over my shoulder to shout to her brother.

'It's all right,' she yelled. 'Mummy isn't angry.'

There was no movement from Oli's room. He still wasn't sure if he'd got away with such a mess.

'I've asked if we can have another bath tomorrow, Oli,' his hopeful sister shouted. 'Can we, Mummy? I'd love another bath just like that one.'

She looked at me as I held her. Her eyes were bright with happiness.

'I think we'll have to see about that, Han,' I said and smiled at her.

CHAPTER SEVEN

Everyone is Equal

❀

It is June now and Phoebe was five last week so we had a party for her at home. She was so excited about it she almost bounced off the ceiling and started running around yelling as soon as she saw the balloons Mum had blown up and the cake, crisps and chocolate on the kitchen table.

I'd helped Mum get everything ready while Phoebe was at school. I wasn't very well last week and had been in bed a lot because I had too much fluid in me, which is what happens when my heart isn't pumping fast enough and my liver is suffering. So I got up late on Phoebe's birthday, helped Mum lay the table and make a trifle and then went back to bed again. Mum only has to tell me to lie down when I'm excited, like on Dad's birthday. Otherwise I know when I need to go to bed, just like I know what to do with my medicines.

Mum started letting me take them when I came out of hospital after the pacemaker because I wanted to know what I was taking and when. In the morning I take captopril, furosemide, carvedilol, spironolactone, digoxin, aspirin and Q10; at lunchtime it's captopril and furosemide; then in the evening I finish with captopril, furosemide, carvedilol, spironolactone and Q10. I know it sounds complicated but it's not when you get used to it.

I got up again when Phoebe, Lucy and Oli came back from school and the party started. I'd bought Phoebe a ra-ra skirt, some sweets and a dot-to-dot colouring book, and Mum and Dad had given her a pink keyboard and an art fun pack. Dad was away working so he wasn't there but Grandma and Grandad came and we had Phoebe's party in the lounge. By 5.30 p.m., though, I felt really tired again and had to go back to bed.

I didn't feel like doing anything much for a few days more after that. If I get ill then our GP, Dr Knight, usually comes to see me and talks to Mum about giving me a bit more furosemide or something. If it's really bad then I have to go into Hereford Hospital to see the doctor who's looked after me ever since I was little. His name is Dr Meyrick and he's really nice.

Now I'm out of bed again because I'm feeling a bit better, and yesterday I went up to the horse field with Lucy. Before my heart got worse we used to go together a lot more. We'd wash the ponies, play in the fields in the long grass and then wait for Mum to come and see what we'd done – she was always surprised when the ponies were immaculate. Lucy could be a bit annoying back then because she'd run off to play so I'd have to tell her to come back and finish helping me. But now she does the ponies on her own most of the time and even gets up really early on school mornings to do them if I'm ill and Mum can't leave the house.

Yesterday, though, I felt OK and helped Lucy a bit as she washed Mr Minty with special shampoo. It's purple and we sponged it on before rubbing out the grass stains on his coat and washing the shampoo off. It worked really well and by the time we'd finished Mr Minty looked as white as white can be again. I liked doing it because Mum was pleased with us and we got to get away from Phoebe who's been mad ever since her birthday. It was also good to be out of the house because I'd been there for too long. I like the freedom of being outside where there are no walls, you can breathe in fresh air and the fields run on for ever. I'd run up and down them a hundred times if I could. I like the sound, the light, the noise of grass crunching under your feet as you walk.

It was good to go out with Lucy too because I'm friends with all my family but especially her. Even though Lucy's three years younger than me, we're not that different and we're good mates. Sometimes I argue with her and Oli, though, because they wind me up when they keep coming into my bedroom, which is really annoying. On the days when I'm ill, Phoebe always seems to want something and Oli and Lucy start fighting because they know Mum's with me so it's a good time to get away with it. When that happens I wish they weren't there because then Mum could spend the whole day with me. If I'm feeling poorly I like her near me and although I know a lot of her attention goes on me I still sometimes wish I didn't have to share her or Dad with my brother and sisters.

Phoebe's too young to understand what's wrong with me and I think Oli and Lucy find it hard to imagine being in my place. Sometimes I wonder if they think it's easy being ill because I get things I want like my own TV. I had a massive old one before but saved up my pocket money to buy a flat screen because I spend so much time watching stuff in bed. I thought I'd have enough to buy one so I asked Dad to take me into town to help me pick. But then I saw how much the televisions cost and realised I didn't have enough. Luckily Dad said he'd lend me some extra as long as I saved up to pay him back later.

That's the kind of thing that makes Oli and Lucy jealous, though, and I could tell when we got home that they wished they had a TV too. But although I know they think my life is easy, I wish I could ride as well as Lucy or go on the school bus like Oli does every day. I'd like to go out and do stuff like that but can't because I don't have enough power in my heart to keep a bike going or get on and off a bus every day. I wish I was like my brother and sister, but we're different.

It's good in some ways because the world would be very boring if everyone was the same. But sometimes it's hard and they tell me I get everything I want when we argue. When they do that I want to tell them that having to make all these decisions isn't easy, having to be in hospital and missing my friends is awful and I try my hardest not to be spoiled even though they think I am. But I don't say all that so instead I just tell myself I can't run around and do the things they can so I need stuff to entertain me.

Don't get me wrong. Oli and Lucy aren't any nastier to me than I am to them. I wind them up all the time by hiding their things or annoying them in other ways. But I can't help being ill,

I can't stop all this and they don't know both sides of the coin like I do: being well and going to school, being ill and lying in bed. So when they get annoyed I have to tell myself that they don't mean it and it isn't my fault I was made like this.

The only other thing that really gets to them is when they think I'm not getting told off as much as they are. They're right because I don't but it's got nothing to do with being ill. I'm just not as naughty as they are. I was sent to my bedroom a lot when I was eleven but I'm not so bad now I'm thirteen. I'm growing up.

I listened to the sound of the children downstairs. Nearly six months pregnant with my fourth child, I was suffering from very bad morning sickness and had also started getting labour pains a week ago before being given drugs to stop them. Now I was in bed resting and could hear Hannah downstairs as she shooed her brother and sister around to make sure they got ready for school.

In the two years since her central line had been removed Hannah had grown stronger, and now, as she approached her ninth birthday, the five-year anniversary of her remission was just months away. Once I'd have thought it impossible that such a milestone could go unmarked. But the anniversary's power had slowly ebbed as the years had passed and Hannah had remained well. Her blood tests had been consistently clear and her heart function had risen. She had got stronger and the hope that she would one day lead a normal life had bedded itself inside me and already started to take root. Our life was moving on and our family would soon take on a new shape.

At first I'd worried that my morning sickness was making it impossible for me to do as much as usual around the house. But I'd soon realised that it meant Hannah did more for herself, and I was glad because I wanted her to grow to be as confident and independent as Oli and Lucy were.

They had had to start learning from a young age because as much as I'd tried to make sure that Oli and Lucy got enough of my attention, I'd had no choice but to trust them to do things. They had learned a great deal because of it and could take Hannah's medications to her by the age of five. Counting the pills into their hands, I'd tell them to count them back into Hannah's and listen to make sure they did. When they started school, I left them to clean their own teeth and faces – Oli standing beside Lucy at the basin as she peered over the side of the sink – while I gave Hannah her morning medications and cooked the breakfast.

It meant they started to test, learn and trust their limits early and it pleased me because I wanted something different for them to the restricted childhood I'd had. Hannah had taught me to see new ways of being a parent and embrace, instead of fear, them so Lucy's independent streak had showed itself by the age of four when she got sick of Oli putting lopsided bunches into her hair and taught herself to do it, while her brother's trustworthiness was apparent when I started letting him walk her to school. We were lucky because Whitbourne was a quiet village with little traffic but I also knew that even at the age of seven Oli would make sure his sister followed the pavement on the four-minute walk.

I rejoiced in their achievements: watching them grow and spending time with them. We went riding, I took Oli to football practice or drew pictures with Lucy. But some of my happiest moments came when I wasn't physically with them. Instead I would watch their heads disappearing through a field of long grass and it made me happy to know they felt completely free.

I knew I was very different to many mothers and I remember a conversation outside the school gates about morning routines which left both me and the woman I was talking to a little startled – me because of how much she did for her children, she because of how little I seemed to do in comparison. But while I was careful not to overload Oli and Lucy with responsibility, I had learned that children are capable of a lot if they are allowed to be.

Sometimes of course it all backfired on me, like the day Lucy decided to ride her tiny white Shetland pony Snoopy into the kitchen. I was upstairs when I heard a crash and raced down to find Hannah looking up from the sofa in the kitchen where she always rested at Lucy who was sitting on her pony a couple of feet away.

'What on earth are you up to?' I screeched as I caught sight of a big pile of dung on the kitchen floor.

'Lucy brought Snoopy to see me because I can't get to the field to visit him,' Hannah said.

The girls started giggling uncontrollably as I stared at them.

'Well, I think you need to take him back there,' I said and Lucy sighed as she turned the pony towards the French windows leading out into the garden.

His hooves clipped across the floor as she rode out and I stared after her in wonder and horror, wondering what my children would get up to next.

But while they knew they had freedom – and sometimes tested it to the limits – they were also aware of their responsibilities and the few strict lines that couldn't be crossed which included going to bed on time, always being polite and doing what I asked when I asked. I wanted their home to be full of respect, love and laughter, and I hope that's what I gave them.

Now I listened as I heard the front door open and the children clatter outside.

'Bye, Mummy,' Lucy yelled.

I couldn't even raise my head off the pillow to say goodbye, and I lay still in bed until Hannah appeared at the door a few minutes later.

'I walked Oli and Lucy to the garden gate and watched them to the end of the road,' she told me as she stood by the bed. 'Now would you like some water, Mummy?'

'Yes please, Han,' I murmured gratefully.

I lay my head back down as I listened to her walking back downstairs. I was pleased: Hannah was becoming independent. It was just the way it should be.

~

My third daughter Phoebe was born sixteen weeks prematurely and weighed just 1lb 9oz. My strongest memory of her birth was moments after she was delivered by emergency caesarean when someone asked what I'd like the doctors to do with her, as if there was any doubt.

'Anything and everything you can,' I replied.

I'd wanted to fight my body, to force it to keep my baby safe inside me, after I went into labour. But I couldn't stop what was happening and was rushed by ambulance to Bristol for an emergency delivery. By the time I woke up from the anaesthetic, Phoebe had been taken to intensive care and the nurses told me to rest. But I had to see her and asked Andrew to push me to the baby unit in a wheelchair. A row of identical incubators lined each side of the room, but something made me stop at the second cot on the right. I couldn't see a name on it but knew that Phoebe was inside.

Staring into it, my heart turned as I saw her for the first time – she was so small that the tiny teddy bear lying in her crib dwarfed her. Just six inches long, her eyes were still fused shut and she had no fingernails, hair or eyebrows. But as I looked at Phoebe I felt a familiar feeling rise up inside me – an intertwining of love and protection so strong that it almost took my breath away. Once again, one of my children was fighting for her life and I had to do all I could to help her survive.

The doctors had warned me that the risk of a brain haemorrhage or fatal infection was very high in such a premature baby. But the same instinct which had awoken when Hannah fell sick guided me again now. Things as simple as breathing and eating were hard for Phoebe, and because she was so premature I was not yet producing milk properly. So I would collect it, drop by drop, because all she needed was one millilitre an hour in her tiny stomach. Her lungs, like those of many premature babies, were also undeveloped and so I would lift her out of the incubator and sit for hour after hour with her lying naked against my bare chest because I knew such kangaroo care could help a baby's breathing. Watching her nestle against me, with a ventilator tube up her nose, an oxygen probe on her toe and a nasogastric tube for feeding, Phoebe looked as if she was hovering on the edges of our world and I marvelled at just how strong the will to live can be.

For six weeks I lived in a bubble with her – focused once again on my sick child as everything else was forgotten. Andrew and his parents had picked up everything at home and Phoebe was all that mattered now. When the children came in to see us, they would look in wonder at their tiny sister lying in the incubator. But while Oli and Lucy seemed happy to meet their new sister, Hannah was a little scared of the intensive care unit at first. I wondered if it awoke deeply buried memories, but gradually she started to help me when she came in for a visit and forgot whatever might have been stirred inside her.

'I can do it,' she'd say as I went to make sure the tubes connected to Phoebe were lying comfortably or to turn her every twenty minutes to even out the pressure on her tiny skull.

'Are you sure, Han?'

'Yes.'

Then I would watch as she reached into the incubator, her small hands holding her sister gently as she moved her.

Day by day, Phoebe got stronger until she was well enough to be moved to Worcester and I had to leave her at night. I hated not being there but Andrew had once again had so much time off work that I had return home to do the school run and pack lunch boxes, hang clothes on the line and prepare food. But my mind was constantly with Phoebe as I thought of her in that strange hospital so far away, and I drove to see her twice a day between school runs.

Hannah came with me for every visit and would sit quietly as I fed Phoebe, watching her for signs of distress or illness, praying each day that she would continue to be well. Slowly I realised I had been given another miracle as Phoebe grew stronger – the second of my children who had clung to life but was gradually filled with it once again.

By the time Phoebe arrived at Hereford for the final weeks of her three-and-a-half-month hospital stay, she was off the ventilator and the nasogastric tube. She was so near now that I could drive in to breastfeed her five times a day, and by the time she came home she weighed 4lb 1oz – small certainly in comparison to my other children, but well and healthy. I could only give thanks again that I had been given this gift.

At first I wondered if it might unsettle Hannah when Phoebe came home because it had been just the two of us during the school day for so long. But she relished the chance to help and be an older sister – fetching nappies and bottles, or making me a cup of tea which she'd bring as I breastfed.

I soon realised, though, that things couldn't stay as they had been for so long. As time had passed I'd been thinking about sending Hannah back to school – undecided about whether it would be too much physically but knowing it would be good for her in other ways. Now the decision had been taken out of my hands because I just didn't have enough time to educate Hannah and look after a new baby.

Six months after Phoebe was born we moved to a village between Hereford and Worcester called Burley Gate, where Hannah started primary school. She attended gradually – building up from mornings to full days – and was ready to start the school year properly by September 2005. It felt right that Hannah's life was changing, and while she knew there were still limits to what she could do because of her heart –

she would never run races or ride horses, for instance – she seemed to have accepted them.

More and more now I could live without worrying over every tiny cough and cold she had. Each time we saw Hannah's doctors they told us that her heart function was stable, and over the years it had even increased to around 25 per cent. Hannah's body was coping, and when we went for a check-up every four months it was a question of monitoring rather than increasing her treatment. Looking into the future, I imagined Hannah as one of those Victorian ladies who led quiet but fulfilled and happy lives, taking regular medication but needing no other treatment.

As she took her first steps into the world at school, I realised just how much Hannah's illness had shaped her character. She and I had slipped into an easy routine at home but now Hannah revealed a determination that I'd never seen before as she started testing her limits. She had not seen the world in the same way as Oli and Lucy or challenged her physical limits as they had, but she was fearless about expressing herself in classroom discussions and could be equally as implacable in her actions when she'd made her mind up. One memorable day I gave each of the children money to buy Christmas presents for each other, but Hannah didn't look as Oli and Lucy hunted the shelves.

'Can't you find anything you like?' I asked as she walked behind me.

'No.'

'Well, there must be something.'

'I'm not going to look.'

'Why?'

'Because I'm not going to get Oli and Lucy anything.'

'Why?'

'They were mean to me yesterday.'

'That doesn't seem very fair if they're buying you presents,' I said.

'I don't care,' she replied. 'I'm not getting them anything.'

I stopped to look at Hannah, knowing that if I chose to fight this battle with her then I would have to see it through.

"It's Christmas, Han,' I said. 'I don't think you should worry about what they said yesterday. Oli and Lucy are going to buy you something and you should get them a present too.'

'No.'

'Well then, I'll have to tell them to put back their things for you. It's not fair if they buy you presents and you don't get them something. Is that what you want?'

Hannah stayed silent, and it was the same during arguments when she refused to back down. However much I tried to reason with her, Hannah wouldn't budge if she believed she was in the right, and while I could usually convince her brother and sister to apologise, there was nothing I could do to change her mind. Inwardly I smiled at her stubborn nature, which was so like mine, but outwardly I had to try and temper it, however much of a losing battle I knew I was fighting.

I cherished her strength because Hannah could so easily have been a frightened and hesitant child. But her illness had forged her character in ways that I was only just beginning to understand. All the months and years of doctors and nurses asking her to do things she didn't necessarily like had made Hannah far more definite than most children about what she was – and wasn't – prepared to do. She knew her own mind in a way which astounded me and had an utter self-belief in what she thought she was right. It was her form of rebellion, born out of a necessity to believe in herself when she was plunged into an experience that no one could share with her – Hannah had fought for her life and it had taught her a great deal.

Soon there would be mornings when she would refuse to take her tablets and once again I knew it was a battle that I couldn't fight because I would certainly lose it, however much I didn't want to. Of course I tried to reason with her and sometimes became so desperate that I'd resort to almost frightening her into taking the medicines as I told her how much her heart needed them. But Hannah wouldn't say a word as she sat silently with her lips clamped shut. Her strength of will was frustrating and astounding in equal measure.

Hannah wasn't the only one, though, who had been deeply affected by her illness – Oli and Lucy's school reports often mentioned how considerate and patient they were with less able children, and both of them had learned well how to stick up for someone who stood out. Oli's best friend was a boy who other children often made fun of because he had mild learning difficulties. But Oli liked him for what he could do, didn't care about the things he couldn't, and that was that.

Lucy was equally accepting, but where her brother was calm and laid back she had fire in her belly. After also starting at a new school, she made friends with a girl who was picked on because she was smaller than the other children. Lucy was outraged and burned with a sense of injustice so great that one day she ended up in a tussle with another pupil and got sent to the headmaster's office after defending her friend. I knew she shouldn't have done it but admired her courage. I wanted all my children to live their lives bravely and know that no matter our differences, weaknesses or strengths, everyone was equal.

I got up and walked to the living room window to stare down the road for the hundredth time. It was 4.30 p.m. on an average October afternoon – dusk was falling and Oli and Lucy were watching TV after coming home from school. But this was an extraordinary day and one which had made me anxious and overjoyed in equal measure.

Hannah had started at secondary school a few weeks before in a large village about a fifteen-minute drive from our home, and it was a huge milestone. After completing a year at primary school, she'd moved onto the next stage and was blossoming. She'd made friends and was full of stories about them. School discos, GCSEs, sleepovers and becoming a teenager were all rushing closer and closer. Sometimes I wanted to pinch myself when I thought back to just a few years before when life had been so uncertain. Now it finally felt dependable again with three children at school and two-year-old Phoebe growing up fast.

Each step Hannah had taken into her new life was important but today felt especially so because it was the first time she'd gone on the school bus. Ever since she'd started back at primary school, I'd either driven Hannah or walked in with her. Now, after six weeks at big school, she'd decided she wanted to go on the bus just like everyone else.

I knew the travelling might tire her. Still on about six types of heart medication which she took in three doses over the day, Hannah could get run down if she did too much. But she wanted to be the same as her classmates and I could remember how that felt. It was the most important thing to her, just as it should be. After all these years she was finally becoming her own person.

'I'll walk you to the bus stop and then pick you up when you get back,' I'd told her as we talked about it.

'No, Mum,' she insisted. 'I don't want you to meet me. The other mums don't go to the bus. My friends just walk home. Why can't I?'

I looked at her, knowing I had to let her stretch herself just as Oli and Lucy had been doing for years. This wasn't about Hannah's limits but testing mine and letting her go, trusting her to be as responsible as I knew deep down that she could be. I had spent years trying to balance Hannah's, Oli's and Lucy's different needs and show that all of them were equally important. Now I had to let go and allow Hannah to be like any other child of her own age.

'Will you let me walk you there on the first morning if I promise not to meet the bus again?' I asked.

'All right, but then will you let me get home a bit late?'

'Why?'

'Because I want to go to the shop.'

So Hannah and I had made a deal and this morning I'd walked her to the bus stop and watched as she got on. I knew she was looking forward to telling her school friends about her journey and she smiled at me before waving as the bus pulled away. My heart tugged a little as I watched her go.

Now I glanced at my watch and told myself I had to do something other than stare out of the window. I walked into the kitchen and put on the kettle as I wondered where Hannah was. The bus would have dropped her off about twenty minutes ago, more than enough time to get to the shop and back. Should I go and look for her? Would she be OK?

Suddenly I heard the thud of the front door slamming and a bag being dropped on the hallway floor. Footsteps padded down towards the kitchen and Hannah appeared at the door. I wanted to run at her and start firing questions. Instead, I poured some water onto a tea bag and tried to look relaxed.

'Hi, Mum,' she said as she walked in.

'Hello, darling.'

'What's for tea?'

'Spaghetti bolognaise.'

'Great.'

She sat down at the kitchen table and I gave her a mug of tea.

'Thanks,' she said.

'So how was the bus, Han?' I asked as I sat down.

'Fine.'

Just like that. One word. Nothing more. What did fine mean? Who had she talked to? Had she got a seat on the bus?

'Did you get to school OK?'

'Yes.'

'Did you get back?'

She looked at me in exasperation.

'Of course I did! I'm here, aren't I, Mum?'

'So where have you been?' I asked, unable to keep silent a moment longer.

'To the shop, like I said.'

She pulled a white paper bag out of her pocket.

'I bought us all some sweets. Where are Oli and Lucy?'

She picked up her mug and walked out of the kitchen. I smiled to myself as I heard her call her brother and sister.

CHAPTER EIGHT

The Right to Choose

❀

I know most kids wouldn't say this but I loved secondary school. I LOVED it. I wasn't sure about primary because I hadn't been for so long and all I could remember was a teacher shouting at me when I didn't do my homework right. I hadn't seen *High School Musical* back then and so the only other stuff I knew was what Lucy had told me. She'd said she liked the food but that didn't tell me much because Lucy likes any kind of food.

So I was nervous when I went back to school because I only knew one girl there. Her name was Becky and she was in Year 6 – the one above me, which means a lot when you're at primary school. But during my first break time Becky asked if I wanted to join in the game she was playing with Jennifer, Ruth and Grace and then helped me find my classroom, so I realised school wasn't going to be that bad.

The teacher I really liked was called Mr Burrell. He was quite round, tall and always knew how to make things fun because he'd been a theatre director and could turn anything into a joke during lessons. But just as I was getting used to primary and made a friend called Julia, I had to go on to secondary school, so I felt nervous again.

St Mary's seemed massive on my first day there – full of kids rushing around and Year 8, 9, 10 and 11s who all knew each other. This time I really was on my own and felt weird in my brand new uniform – a blazer with electric blue, yellow and white stripes, a white shirt with long sleeves and navy skirt. I'd never worn anything like it and some of the other girls' skirts looked really short so I wondered if mine was wrong.

But then I met Simone and everything changed because I realised that people who are really different can be good friends. Simone is bubbly and I'm quieter, she's tall and I'm short, she looks fifteen, I look younger because I'm little. But there was one important thing which was the same – we both laughed at things we're not supposed to, which happened all the time because Simone is a nutter.

She is my true friend. Simone understands everything, doesn't question me about things I don't want to talk about, and if I don't get to school then she phones me up to tell me what's going on. For a long time I wished I could have a best friend – someone to muck around and talk about normal stuff with, a proper, 100 per cent friend who I could tell secrets to. That's what Simone is, and when I was at school I learned that if you look after your friends they'll look after you. It's like in *The White Giraffe* where the girl has to move to Africa after her parents die and she becomes friends with a giraffe. I know a giraffe's not the same as Simone but it's not that different either because the girl and the giraffe trust each other, just like Simone and I.

The other people we made friends with were Becky, Brigitta, Laura, Kelcea and Zoe, and they're all brilliant too. Every morning before school we'd sit on a window sill near our form rooms and chat about random things like *Twilight*, which boy was most annoying, homework and stuff. It was great but what I liked most was that no one knew about my heart. I'd told Simone a bit but otherwise people didn't know until they saw me on the news after I said no to the transplant and the secret was out.

But when I first started at St Mary's only the teachers knew and my friends just saw me as one of them. All I could think was 'Great!' I was at school full-time, not taking too many pills (I even forgot to take them sometimes) and I didn't get too tired. In fact I couldn't sit down much because I was such a fidget. It was so good being normal that I even liked getting on the bus even though I didn't like the drivers after one of them had a massive go at me when I gave him my fare and he suddenly told me it had gone up. Luckily I had 20p to give him but he still told me off.

'Make sure you've got the right money next time,' he said and made me feel bad even though I hadn't done anything wrong.

I didn't know what to say as my friend Emily tried to stick up for me.

'She didn't know, it was an accident,' she told the driver.

Then he told her to be quiet and I couldn't believe it. He was so rude.

But apart from the bus drivers, I loved going to school and was up for everything except PE. The other kids made me laugh a lot, like the time a boy called Tom was mucking around and a teacher who's a right old witch said we all had to come back for a lunchtime detention. Luckily, I was held back after the lesson before lunch to help my form tutor with the chairs so there was only fifteen minutes of the detention left by the time I had finished. So I asked myself: lunch or detention – which was more important? I knew the answer right away: lunch, of course.

The other best bits of school were:

- Someone blowing up their oven in cookery class. The teacher had to use the fire extinguisher on the flames. I can't remember what was cooking, maybe flapjacks or ham and cheese muffins, but somehow someone set their oven alight and everyone really laughed.

- My maths teacher, Mr Robinson. I'd always hated maths and he was really nice so it got a bit easier. Teachers are really important because they can make you like a subject or not.

- When people mucked around and played up so we missed a bit of a lesson. I liked watching other people be naughty.

- My first sleepover at Simone's when I was in Year 7. I hadn't been on a sleepover before and wondered what would happen if Simone decided she didn't like me. But it was brilliant.

- History lessons with Mr Carter because he made us laugh. Once we had a lesson about Roman architecture and ended up singing the *Bob the Builder* theme tune. How random is that?

But if I had to pick one best bit about school then it would be my friends because it's when I finally learned how important they are and realised that, although I love my family, everyone needs people of their own age to mix with. It scared me a bit to go up to people I didn't know and chat to them at first but then I made friends and really appreciated them.

That's the main reason why I hated it so much when I got ill again. I was normal, I was at school, I had mates and sleep-overs, I was like everyone else. And then one day I went to school in the morning and by that night I was ill in hospital again. It's hard to explain how it made me feel but hospital is where everything that's bad has ever happened to me so it wasn't good.

I sometimes look back and wonder how I didn't see clouds gathering on the horizon again. Maybe it was because my focus was on the here and now instead of the distance, but more likely it was the fact that I thought my concerns about Hannah's health were misplaced. In the first few months of 2007 fear had flickered at the back of my mind like a crow wheeling on a distant skyline after she'd started complaining of stomach ache and feeling tired. But blood tests, chest and abdominal X-rays were all fine and I didn't stop to consider that Hannah's heart might be worsening because she had been so well for so long. Then came a phone call in the middle of an ordinary day which taught me for the second time that life can fall apart in one sentence.

Andrew had taken Hannah to the GP earlier that day after she'd fallen unwell at school. Now they were at Hereford Hospital where Hannah had collapsed.

'They think it's her heart,' he said, his voice clipped with fear.

Another car journey made too quickly, another dash through hospital corridors, until I reached Hannah who was lying semi-conscious in a bed. I told myself it was a temporary problem, a virus or infection that would be quickly resolved. That was all it would be – nothing serious or debilitating. Hannah was finally moving through life instead of waiting, always waiting, to be strong enough to live it.

But Andrew's face was stricken as Dr Meyrick, the consultant who'd known Hannah since the first night she fell ill with leukaemia, told us that she was dangerously sick. Her heart was enlarged and not beating powerfully enough, which meant she was struggling to get enough oxygen. Vital organs like her kidneys and liver were also suffering.

'Hannah is in sudden and acute heart failure,' he said gravely. 'I've sent a copy of her scan to Birmingham and she is going to be transferred to their intensive care unit immediately. She needs intravenous drugs to act directly on her heart. Time is of the essence.'

He could not tell us why Hannah's heart had so suddenly deteriorated, and Andrew and I could only watch numbly as she was put into an ambulance. Had we been careless with our happiness? Taken too much for granted? For so long I'd been ready for this moment, almost expecting it even. But years had passed and I'd trusted them, I'd believed Hannah was safe again and now I knew I should never have been so complacent.

Andrew went home to arrange for someone to look after Oli, Lucy and Phoebe while I got into the car to follow the ambulance up the motorway. As I watched its lights flash blue in front of me, I remembered the last time we'd made this journey when Hannah was small. Now I could feel the world closing down to her and me once again, just as it had all those years ago. Soon we would be flung back into the familiar rush of hospital emergency, a landscape where the horizon could shift at any second. Hannah's life was in danger for a second time, and as adrenalin coursed around my body I knew I must prepare to fight with her. I would not lose her. I could not lose her.

The doctor stood beside me as I sat by Hannah's bed. He was holding an anaesthetic consent form which I needed to sign to give permission for Hannah to undergo surgery. For the past three days medics at Birmingham Children's Hospital had been trying to stabilise her after an echocardiogram had revealed that Hannah's heart function had dropped to just ten per cent. Her liver and kidneys were also failing and she needed a central line inserted to make sure she got enough of the drug called Dobutamine which was keeping her alive now.

It acted like adrenaline to stimulate Hannah's heart contractions, but getting enough of the Dobutamine into her body was difficult. Hannah's heart was pumping so weakly that her veins weren't being opened by sufficient blood flow and they kept collapsing even when the Dobutamine was finally administered because the drug was so strong. She also needed a range of drugs to counteract other symptoms and deal with the side effects of so many medications.

Still semi-conscious, Hannah had nevertheless become increasingly distressed as the days had passed. Allergic to local anaesthetic, she felt every needle as it punctured her body – sometimes as many as eight at one time sticking into her hands and feet – just as pain shot through her when an inch-long cut was made in her elbow to thread a long line under her skin. It travelled via her armpit along a vein to her heart but the site went septic within twenty-four hours as the Dobutamine burned a hole the size of a one-pence piece into the crook of her elbow. Now the only option left for effectively administering the Dobutamine was a central line, just like the one Hannah had had as a child to deliver her chemotherapy drugs.

But the anaesthetic she would need to put the line in place was a huge risk for someone whose heart was so dangerously weak. Standing next to me, the anaesthetist bent down as I took the form and he silently traced his finger along a line of words. My eyes followed his finger as each word leapt off the page: 'This procedure can result in death.' My hand quivered for a moment as I held the pen before pressing it onto the paper to sign my name. Hannah's heart failure had not been caused by an infection that could be cured in a few days with antibiotics and neither was it a problem that could be solved with immediate surgery. The doctors did not know why her health had so suddenly deteriorated but the only thing keeping her alive now was the Dobutamine. She needed the central line.

Soon Hannah was taken down to theatre and once again all I could do was wait as I forced myself to let the minutes tick by. I thought of the memories we'd spent so many happy years together collecting: Hannah giggling as she sat in a bath full of bubbles, all the children plunging their hands into pots of paint, Snow White bending down to give her a kiss, Hannah's smile as she'd arrived back from a trip to Lourdes just a few weeks ago. It was the place of miracles, and to me Hannah had been one for so long: well and happy, she was living a life she'd so nearly lost.

Now I felt disorientated as I stared up at the grey hospital walls and my memories melted away. Every familiar point I'd built up around us, every dependable thing we had learned to trust had disappeared again. I'd always known that the heart damage caused by the chemotherapy was irreversible and had quietly accepted that Hannah may not live as long as a completely healthy child. But I'd dared to imagine her growing into adulthood, and now nothing was sure.

Slowly I counted down the thirty minutes that I'd been told she would be in theatre. Time slid by as I stared at my watch, and it was two and a half hours before the surgeon finally came to tell me that she was waking up.

'We had to put the line into her neck because of the scarring from older procedures,' he told me. 'It's now running across her chest wall, which might be a bit more uncomfortable, and her veins were also very narrow so it was a bit tricky at times. She was poorly on the table but she's waking up now.'

I knew enough to read between the doctor's reassurances.

'Was there an emergency?'

'Yes.'

My whole body jolted as I heard those words. Hannah must have had a cardiac arrest, and although I knew this was not uncommon in heart patients undergoing surgery, terror gripped me as the doctor started to leave.

'She's fine now, Mrs Jones,' he said softly as he opened the door. 'We've done what we had to and she's through it.'

I forced myself to take a deep breath as he left the room. I had to remember what Hannah had taught me, what we had lived during all these years – to be in the moment, to live each one with hope, however dark the road ahead seemed.

❦

Machines clicked and beeped as Hannah lay on the bed. A doctor was standing beside her and I tensed as I heard the crackle of a sterilised needle pack being opened. Even though the central line was in place now, Hannah still required a cocktail of other drugs to keep her stable, and the doctor was going to insert a needle into the top of her foot to give her saline.

'No!' Hannah moaned as the needle slid underneath her skin and her body tensed in pain.

'That's it now, darling,' I said. 'It's all over.'

But even as I comforted Hannah and the saline bag was suspended from a drip stand, I knew she would soon need another needle inserted. Once the fluid had gone into her system, Hannah's heart would not be able to pump it properly to her weakened kidneys. She would then need albumin to suck the saline through her system before a third needle was inserted to give her furosemide, a drug to help her kidneys pass it out of her body.

It was like a macabre merry-go-round of symptoms, relief, new symptoms and more relief that Hannah was forced to endure each day. Just as she had so many years before, Hannah was paying a high price for the treatment which was saving her life – an endless juggling act between drugs as we waited to see how she would respond.

'Don't let them,' she'd say softly, as a nurse or doctor came to put another needle in. 'Please, Mummy.'

'But they have to,' I would reply, hardly knowing if it made sense any more when I saw how much pain she was in. 'It won't take long and it will make you feel better, Han.'

Then her eyes would close and doubts would fill me as she fell into a troubled sleep. How long could her body cope with this? And, more importantly, how long could her spirit?

Hannah did not have to put into words how much she hated being back in hospital. As days turned into a week and the Dobutamine kept her heart beating, she began to be more wakeful, but her distress hung around her like a shadow. Her eyes were full of disbelief – lifeless, as if shutters had gone down inside, as she struggled to understand how she'd been well one minute and so sick the next. The life she'd been living to the full after so many years of waiting had been snatched away and every fibre in her was straining against this theft.

But the doctors had no choice other than to keep juggling the drugs because it was clear that Hannah could not cope without the Dobutamine. Any change to her dosage – even a decrease of just half a millilitre over twenty-four hours – would make her heart gallop as it tried to beat, her breathing become shallow and her kidneys start to shut down as fluid collected in her tissues. As I watched her struggle, I knew just how fragile Hannah's grip on life was.

When the dosage was increased again she slowly became more alert, but every touch or movement seared into her as the doctors monitored vital signs and gave drugs, the nurses changed dressings and tried to soothe skin raw from needles. All her senses were heightened as her body fought, and Hannah would moan if a light shone too brightly or cry if someone walked into her room and spoke too loudly. Even the sound of a bin being emptied in a corridor outside was enough to unsettle her, and she didn't like to be touched because her skin was painful. Her room had to be dark and quiet, a cocoon in which she fought to live.

It was just the two of us again, and although I knew it pained Andrew to be separated from us again, the ease with which we had all slipped once again into our 'emergency' routine after so many years almost scared me – Andrew looked after Oli, Lucy and Phoebe with his parents while I stayed in hospital with Hannah. So the days passed, bleeding one into another until Hannah began to have moments when she was strong enough to have the television or some music on for a few minutes. She didn't watch or listen properly but at least it was a distraction as she stared blankly at the screen or let the melody wash over her. The only thing which punctured the time were her pleas to go home because in the moments when Hannah felt just a shred more energy she would beg me to take her.

'I want to go home,' she would whisper as tears trickled down her cheeks.

Her words cut into me as I tried to soothe her.

'But you can't, Han. You're poorly. We must wait until you're stronger.'

'Please, Mummy. Please.'

Soon the effort of just a few words would exhaust her and Hannah would fall silent again. But day by day I could sense her despair growing. I could see it in her, feel it hanging in the air around me. Even as she tried to understand why she was back in hospital again, she just couldn't accept it. I saw the questions in her eyes, just as they had been there years before, as she wondered what was being done to her and why. Were old memories being wakened? Experiences do not disappear, memories lie buried inside us like the rings marking a tree's life – hidden from view but part of our very core.

Hannah did not argue or get angry. She was too weak to do anything other than retreat into herself, but her silence told me everything I needed to know. This was supposed to be her time now – time to go to school and make friends, time to make mistakes and be a teenager, time to grow into her world and create a new one for herself as she moved towards adulthood. Had I been wrong to believe that she could?

Watching her suffer made me feel desperate and powerless. At least when Hannah was a small child there were hospital play leaders to cajole her into a smile and she could be soothed by something as simple as the sound of my voice reading a fairy tale. But she was on the verge of becoming a young woman now and sometimes rage at the injustice of what was happening to her coursed through my veins. I wanted to rail against it if Hannah could not herself.

The water felt warm as it closed around my hands, and I soaked the flannel before wringing it out. Was it soft enough? I'd hunted through every one in the shop to find the softest and would use this just a couple of times before discarding it. It would be too harsh for Hannah's skin after a couple of washes.

I opened out the warm flannel and dabbed at her face with small, light strokes. I would start at her forehead and move down. I had to be quick but not too quick, make sure she was clean but also keep her warm while I washed her.

'It won't take long, darling,' I said softly.

Hannah was lying propped up by pillows. Her neck muscles were so weak now that she could not lift her head for more than thirty seconds without help. Her weight had halved over the past month and her muscles had also wasted as her body fought. Hannah did not have the energy to eat and weighed just a little over three stone now – less than a healthy four-year-old.

A drop of water trickled down the side of her neck and I dabbed it dry. It would feel cold if it collected on her skin, uncomfortable even if unseen.

'I'm going to do your mouth now, Han,' I told her as I picked up a jar of Vaseline.

I rubbed some gently onto her cracked lips before wrapping cotton wool around the tip of a cotton bud and soaking it in water. The hospital gave me sponges on sticks to use for Hannah's mouth care, but they were too hard. I pulled back her bottom lip, tiny bit by bit, before easing the cotton bud into her mouth to clean it.

When I had finished and her face was clean, I unscrewed the top of a bottle of moisturiser. The sweet smell cut into the clinical hospital air, opening a window onto another world – of perfumes and music, makeup and friends. But Hannah was quiet as I massaged the moisturiser into her skin – increasing the pressure just a little over her forehead and cheeks to relax her. Later I would gently press the pad of her big toe, a moment's focus on a pressure point that I hoped would soothe her.

I lifted the basin of water and walked to the bottom of her bed where I balanced it on a table. Rolling up the sheet and blanket covering Hannah's legs, I left her top half covered to make sure she stayed warm. Over her legs lay one half of a pair of pyjama bottoms that I'd cut in two. Hannah was too weak to get in and out of clothes, and something as small as lying on a crease of fabric was too much for her. But she didn't like it if the doctors pulled back her covers and saw her naked, so I draped clothes across her to make her feel dressed.

I folded one half of the pyjama bottoms to the side before lifting Hannah's foot and rolling it in ever widening circles. This would work the muscles from her knee down, and we tried to do exercises like these twice a day. The joint in her knee looked huge, almost incongruous in her tiny, withered leg as I lay it back down on the towels. Quickly, I washed her leg before covering it up again and moving to the other one which I then exercised and washed.

When her bottom half was clean, I pulled back the blankets covering her from the waist up. Hannah lay listlessly, knowing I had to do this but wanting it finished. She didn't like to be touched more than she had to be so I worked in silence, pulling back the soft cotton top with buttons which lay across her bare chest and washing one arm before lying it down, covering it up and doing the other. I tried not to see her collar bones or rib cage, her breast or hip bones, jutting out angrily from underneath skin so paper thin it looked as if it might break.

When Hannah was finally washed and covered in towels, I moved to the side of the bed to turn her over and do her back.

'It hurts too much,' she whispered.

I thought of the livid red bedsore which had developed on Hannah's coccyx.

I bent to kiss her.

I would stop now.

There was always tomorrow.

As the weeks went on, it became more and more important for Hannah to put on weight because she needed food and calories to give her precious energy. But eating was too much for her most days – it required energy she just didn't have – and she hated the high-calorie build-up soups and drinks she was given so much that a dietician was called in to try and find out if there was anything which might tempt her to eat.

'My mummy knows how I like things,' was all she would say.

I felt increasingly desperate as I sat beside Hannah's bed trying to coax her into eating spoonfuls of food, and eventually it was arranged for me to show a hospital chef how I cooked her food at home in the hope that she might eat it. After going to the local shops to buy the ingredients I usually cooked with, I went to the kitchens and explained how she liked her bolognaise: well-browned mince, no fat and tinned tomatoes.

'No herbs or onion?' the chef asked, a little surprised by the blandness of the meal.

'Nothing else except spaghetti cooked so well you can mash it,' I told him.

Hannah's preference for soft food had stayed with her ever since chemotherapy but she just looked at the meal listlessly later that day when it was delivered to her room.

'Have a taste,' I said. 'Please.'

She opened her mouth without a word and I slid some food into it. She chewed slowly and deliberately, forcing herself to swallow, but kept her mouth closed when I lifted the next spoonful to it.

'Please, Han,' I said softly. 'Just a little bit more?'

'No.'

'But I told the cook exactly how you like it. Have one more bite.'

'No.'

'Please, darling. You need to eat.'

Hannah's eyes began to fill with tears.

'No, Mummy,' she whispered.

'Please?'

'No.'

'But I showed the chef how to make it.'

'It's not the same. You didn't make it at home.'

I didn't force her that day or on many others, but there is one I will never forget or forgive. I had put a spoonful of yoghurt into Hannah's mouth and watched as she didn't swallow. She simply sat and looked at me, her eyes full of questioning and despair. There were moments when it felt as if she was trying to reach inside me, speak to me of the wordless pain and frustration which filled her. Grief clawed at me as I thought of the food in her mouth, her body wasting away. It rushed up and made me almost freeze with desperation until I leaned towards her to pinch her nose shut. I would force her to swallow if I had to. I would not let her die.

But Hannah stared at me as my fingers closed around her nose and I snatched them away. If she couldn't eat then who I was to make her? But if I didn't then how would she survive?

'Will you lift me up, Mummy?' Hannah asked.

I looked out of the window at the bright blue sky which Hannah could only glimpse as she lay in bed. Still too weak to walk or even stand, she longed to see it and I knew that lifting her onto her feet for even just a few seconds would exhaust her. But such tiny moments were precious and so I sat her up before moving her pillows out from behind her.

Sitting down, I wriggled to a kneeling position behind Hannah and put my arms underneath hers. Pushing her up, I knelt on one knee as I raised her to her feet. She felt like a rag doll in my arms, tiny and fragile as I supported her to make sure she didn't have to bear any of her own weight. She leaned against me as she lifted her head to stare out of the window. Drip lines ran from her arms to several bags of medication and fluid hung on stands beside the bed. Her central line poked out of the side of her neck and an oxygen tube ran under her nose. SATS and oxygen monitors were attached to her fingers and toes, and machines beeped softly around us.

Hannah smiled as she looked out of the window.

'It's a lovely day,' she said softly.

The view was mostly just the concrete and bricks of Birmingham's skyline, but Hannah drank in the sight of the world outside. Today it was fine, but she didn't mind what the weather was like: sun made the sky blue, wind sent clouds scudding white across the horizon, rain sent silver drops bouncing like tiny beads of mercury off a flat roof just below her window. She liked to see the world moving outside – particularly on Friday and Saturday nights when the entrance to the police station opposite got busy with lights flashing, cars pulling up and people going in and out.

Soon Hannah had decided that the policemen and women who spent their nights working so hard deserved a treat and asked me to buy them some chocolates. I delivered them one afternoon to a duty sergeant who had looked at me in amazement when I gave him Hannah's present. But to her the giving of a gift was a precious link to life and her desire to be part of it again would almost crackle off her as she slumped back exhaustedly onto her pillows.

Day after day she used what little strength she had to ask me when she could go home, and there was little I could do to reassure her because I just didn't know. The Dobutamine was not a long-term solution for her heart failure because patients were not kept on it indefinitely. But as it continued to keep her alive I told myself that we just had to keep waiting and hoping. Heart failure is not always permanent, and I believed that Hannah could get stronger – just as she had done when her heart first weakened and she was dangerously ill as a child.

But Hannah hated waiting, the endless hours which stretched before her each morning when she woke up, the different sounds and smells, the food at set times, and most of all the countless visits from doctors and nurses – all with a drip or a drain or a medicine to give her. Soon school, just like home, became the focus of her thoughts, and I knew how much she missed her friends.

'I wonder what they're doing today,' she would say. 'Simone and Becky might be in English now.'

Pupils and staff from St Mary's had sent cards and letters which I'd stuck across her walls. Along with those from friends and family, every square inch was covered, and I'd even taken down observation charts to clear more space when new ones arrived. For Hannah it was a vital reminder of all the people who were thinking of her, and she'd been pleased when I'd told her that a teacher was bringing three of her friends up to Birmingham to visit. Hannah was in a room on the high dependency unit and the three girls arrived, bristling with energy and life, to find her lying quietly in bed. Their eyes widened as they saw all the machines that monitored her breathing, pulse and medications.

They left after about an hour and Hannah was too exhausted to talk much – just as she was too tired for most things. If I gave her a Nintendo DS to play with, she would look at it fuzzily before putting it down, unable to focus on the screen because of all the medications; if I offered to paint her toenails she would refuse because she didn't want to be touched any more, too many people were prodding her. Just as she had done when she was a little girl, Hannah retreated into the silent world of her illness.

As the weeks had passed and the doctors continued to juggle Hannah's drugs, I could see she wasn't improving, and so when a month turned into five weeks, then six, I was not surprised when Dr Wright, the kindly cardiologist who had looked after Hannah since she was small, asked to talk to me privately one day. In the long, silent hours by Hannah's bedside I'd thought again and again of the cardiac units I'd once worked on, the intensive care and surgical wards, and knew that if I had nursed a child like her back then, I'd have doubted she could survive. But Hannah was not my patient, she was my child, and I believed in her.

'We have been thinking about more long-term options for Hannah,' Dr Wright said as I sat down with him. 'And we feel her heart function is so low that we must consider the possibility of some other intervention.'

'But surely we should give her a little more time on the Dobutamine?' I asked, knowing even as I spoke that the words tumbling out of my mouth would sound like the desperate hopes of a mother who couldn't see reality for what it was.

Dr Wright was silent for a moment.

'Hannah is very sick,' he said slowly, considering his words carefully. 'We are on the top level of Dobutamine and she is not improving. If we don't do something, Mrs Jones, then she could die, and that is why I wanted to talk to you about the possibility of a heart transplant.'

His words cut into me. A heart transplant? The thought had always been in my mind, ever since that day so many years before when Andrew and I had visited Great Ormond Street. But the possibility had diminished as Hannah grew stronger until I'd hardly thought about it any more. It had seemed so implausible as she got stronger, and surely Hannah might improve again?

'A successful transplant could offer Hannah several more years of healthy life,' Dr Wright continued as I tried to take it all in. 'Patients are now surviving post-operatively for ten or twenty years. This is an area of medicine where advances are being made all the time.'

Even as I listened to what he was saying, I struggled to understand what Dr Wright meant. I'd nursed patients on transplant units before, knew that organs were only given to patients for whom hope was fading. Surely he didn't mean that Hannah was one of them?

'You need to think carefully, Mrs Jones,' Dr Wright continued and I stared at him. 'This is something you should consider. Heart transplants offer children the hope of years of healthy life, and I'm afraid that Hannah will not recover without one.'

The room was silent for a moment. I knew I must speak. I had to say something.

'I'm not sure,' I said finally. 'I need to talk to Hannah.'

Dr Wright didn't reply.

'I know what she wants,' I told him. 'She wants to go home.'

~

The day after I spoke with Dr Wright, he came back to see me.

'I think there might be something else we can try,' he told me. 'Have you heard of a multi-site pacemaker? They are usually given to adult cardiac patients, but we think this device might work for Hannah. There is no guarantee it will, but we have given them to a handful of children and think she might be suitable.'

The pacemaker would work by strengthening the electrical impulses which governed the contractions of Hannah's heart. While most ordinary pacemakers had two wires, a multi-site device contained four – one running into each chamber of the heart – which, unlike other pacemakers, would send out continual electrical impulses. Nothing was sure, but this might help strengthen the muscle tone of Hannah's heart, and although it would take several months until we knew for sure, she could stay on the Dobutamine in the meantime.

As Dr Wright talked, I knew I wanted to do as he suggested. I still felt unsure about a transplant because I wondered if we had quite yet reached this final frontier of hope. A transplant was a place of no return because if it failed there was nothing else that could be done. There were also extra risks for Hannah, just as the doctors had told us long ago, because the anti-rejection drugs could trigger a return of her leukaemia.

But whatever my doubts, I wasn't willing to do nothing and at least the procedure to fit the pacemaker would be far less invasive than a transplant and the post-operative recovery much easier. It would also give us time to think about a transplant while we waited to see what effect the pacemaker had.

Andrew agreed immediately when I phoned to tell him, but both of us knew that the person who would need to be convinced was Hannah. She knew what an operation and another recovery would mean. I thought of her lying in her bed and wondered how I could tell her that she needed surgery, that she wouldn't be able to go home any time soon, see her brother and sisters, smell fresh air or see the sky, stroke Tails McFluff or sleep in her own bed.

Somehow I had to convince her that we must do something, but I wasn't sure what words I would find as I walked into Hannah's room. All I knew as I sat down beside her was that I had to tell her the truth and find out what she thought. If anything was going to help her, then Hannah had to want it to.

'I spoke to Dr Wright today, Han,' I said.

The television was on in the corner of the room and I turned it off as she looked at me.

'You know you're very sick, don't you?' I asked gently. 'And Dr Wright thinks you might need something more to help your heart than the Dobutamine.'

'What do you mean?'

'He thinks you might need an operation.'

I reached out to take her hand. I wanted to feel her skin against mine, feel her with me as we talked about a decision that would change both of our lives.

'What kind?' she asked.

'Either a heart transplant or a pacemaker which is a little box that sits inside your chest and helps your heart to beat.'

'Which one would work better?'

'We don't know, Han. No one can be sure. A heart transplant is a very big operation and doesn't always work but you could live for many years if it did. The doctors aren't certain either that the pacemaker will work but they are willing to try it.'

'How long would I be in hospital if I had a transplant?'

'We can't be certain because it might be a long time if you had to wait for a heart, or it could be just a few weeks.'

She thought about it for a moment before looking at me.

'And how long would I be in hospital if I had the pacemaker?'

'I don't know that either but I think the operation would take less time to recover from.'

'Would I have a scar with both of them?'

'Yes.'

I watched her face, doubts and fears rushing across it as she thought.

'If the pacemaker doesn't work could I have the transplant?'

'Yes.'

'And if the transplant didn't work could I have the pacemaker?'

'No.'

'And what would happen if I didn't have either?'

I faltered for a second before speaking again.

'You could die.'

Recognition flickered in Hannah's eyes. This was the absolute truth. I was hiding nothing.

'I don't want that to happen, Hannah,' I said. 'I want you to get stronger.'

I willed her to trust me, to know that I would do everything in my power to do the best for her as she started crying softly.

'But I don't want another operation,' she sobbed. 'I've had enough. I want to go home.'

'I know, Han.'

I put my arms around her as she buried her head in my chest and the room disappeared in a haze as I listened to Hannah sob. I wanted to stop all this, return our life to how it had been. But I couldn't, and as Hannah pulled away to look at me again our faces were both wet with tears.

'What do you think?' she asked.

'I think we should do what is best for you.'

I could see how strong the urge inside her was to say no to anything else being done. Hannah was tired of hospital and doctors, operations and anaesthetics. She'd had enough.

'Whatever you want is fine by me, Han, but I think we should listen when the doctors say you need more than Dobutamine,' I said gently. 'I know you don't want an operation but I think we should try.'

Hannah lay back on the pillows, almost too weak to say any more.

'I need to know what you think, Han, because if you want to have the pacemaker we can do that, but if you want to have the transplant then that's fine too.'

She looked up at me, her cheeks wet with tears.

'But I don't want either.'

'I know, darling, but I think you have to have one or the other. You are very, very sick and your heart needs help.'

She thought for a moment before speaking again.

'I'll have the pacemaker,' she said softly.

'Are you sure?'

'Yes. Can I go home when it's done?'

'I hope so, Han.'

Days later, Hannah went down to theatre to have the pace-maker fitted by a cardiologist called Dr de Giovanni. Andrew and I had been told the procedure should take about two hours but once again the time dragged by – one hour, one and a half, two hours, two and a half, three hours, four – until Dr de Giovanni came to see us, his face exhausted and sweat dappling his forehead.

'Hannah is out of theatre but I'm afraid we've had a problem,' he said. 'Her veins and arteries are so narrow that we only managed to get the pacemaker box and one of the wires inserted. We still have to place the other three.'

'But how will you do that?' Andrew asked.

Dr de Giovanni told us that he had read about new pace-maker wires which had just been developed abroad for premature babies. He hoped they might fit Hannah's small veins and arteries but they were not yet being manufactured and there was no guarantee the company would be able to provide them. Andrew and I waited nervously as an urgent phone call was made and were relieved when the company agreed to make three wires and fly them over to England with a technician to advise the surgical team on how to insert them.

But it would take a couple of weeks until the wires were ready and for now I had to tell Hannah that she would need another operation. Breaking another piece of bad news worried me. Hannah's trust in me had always felt complete but I wondered if it was being testing to its limits now. She had always known I would protect her but would she ask herself why I was making her stay in a place she hated and undergo surgery that she did not want?

'We can't go home quite yet,' I told her quietly as we sat together. 'The doctors need to do another operation to put some more wires into the pacemaker because they couldn't do it all today.'

'But I want to go home,' Hannah whispered.

'We can't, Han. Not yet.'

'Please, Mummy. Please.'

'I know it's hard, darling, but we have to let the doctors finish what they are doing.'

'No, we don't!'

Anger flared inside her for a moment but quickly disappeared. Her gaze was that of an old soul, staring out from a child's face. It was the same look she had given me so long ago when she had fought for her life the first time, and in moments like those I understood that Hannah had been to places I could never know.

'Please, darling,' I said. 'There's no point in only having half the operation done. We need to let the doctors finish.'

I longed for her to understand that I wasn't ignoring her wishes. I had to find a way to make her understand that once the surgery was done I would do as she wanted.

'I will take you home when the pacemaker is fitted,' I said softly. 'I will make sure we leave here.'

Even as I made the promise, I knew that children on intravenous Dobutamine did not leave hospital. The drug was so powerful that only expertly trained doctors and nurses could administer it. But in that moment I wanted Hannah to believe that I could do as she asked and I wanted to believe that I could do it for her too.

Time stopped for a moment, suspended in the air between us as the seconds stretched into forever until she spoke again.

'OK,' she whispered.

Later that night, Hannah's lung collapsed post-operatively and I watched as she gasped for air while a chest drain was inserted through an incision in her side. As the doctors worked on her, Hannah cried softly and squeezed my hand, fear etched on her face. Whatever it took, I knew I had to take her home. Hannah wanted to live life on her own terms – no one else's.

It took about ten days for the new pacemaker wires to be flown over to the UK, and Hannah was in surgery for several hours as they were fitted. Once again, the operation was gruelling for everyone involved – Hannah, her surgeon, anaesthetist and all the other people who kept her alive throughout it – and when it was finally over she asked once again when she would go home.

At first her doctors were very doubtful about whether she could be discharged on IV Dobutamine. The drug worked directly on her heart so any mistake in administering it could literally mean life or death for Hannah: she could die if her central line got blocked or the solution was too concentrated or weak. Flushing a line containing the drug was also far more complex than anything I'd had to do when she was young because the Dobutamine was so powerful that her condition could deteriorate if she was without it as the line was cleaned. Because of this, I would have to attach her to a second line when I wanted to flush the first one and switch her between the two at exactly the right time to make sure she received a continuous dose of Dobutamine. The drug was also measured in half millilitres and because of all this only specialist nurses and doctors normally attended lines containing it. If Hannah went home from hospital on IV Dobutamine she would be only the second child in the country ever to do so.

The only thing in my favour as I tried to persuade the doctors was my years of experience as a nurse. I had worked in intensive care looking after cardiac patients in the past and knew I could look after Hannah.

'Are you sure?' her doctors would ask as we talked it over. 'You will be completely responsible for her day and night.'

'I know, but I can do it,' I insisted. 'I want to.'

The doubts in their eyes didn't scare me because I was sure of what I had to do. Hannah had had the pacemaker, she'd been given a chance and now she wanted to go home. For her, hospital meant bad memories and pain which she was reminded of every time she put her feet onto lino instead of carpet, watched me fill out a menu card for food she wouldn't eat or heard the endless rumble of a hospital at night instead of silence.

I felt sure that if she was at home she would be happier, eat better and sleep more comfortably – and those things together would give the pacemaker the best possible chance of success. The team at Birmingham had done all we could ask for but I had seen Hannah's will at work throughout her childhood and believed it would sustain her again if we went home. I knew there was a risk that Hannah's body might ultimately be too weak to keep fighting. But I could not let my own fears overrule her wishes. She was more than just a patient. Hannah was a girl on the cusp of becoming a woman and she knew what she wanted.

I took a deep breath as the door closed and I was left in the room alone. A specialist from Great Ormond Street, Dr Wright, nurses and a social worker had just left to go and talk to Hannah again about a transplant. We were due to leave hospital in just a few days after Dr Wright had agreed to let her go home. It was a brave and compassionate decision but first the people looking after Hannah wanted to make sure that she had had no second thoughts about the transplant.

I understood why they needed to. Ever since a transplant had first been mentioned, I'd understood that the weight of medical opinion was behind it. The pacemaker was an unknown and we would have to wait for several months to see if it was effective. Hannah was so weak that no one could be sure she would have that time, and only a successful transplant could offer her a certain solution. It was the choice most people would have made, and Hannah's decision not to was highly unusual.

The doctors had just spoken to Andrew and me about what a heart transplant would mean: the healthy life that children enjoyed after successful surgery and the fact that half of all heart transplant patients were still alive ten years after having surgery. But we were also told that a transplanted heart would not last for ever and most patients suffered from chronic long-term rejection which meant their arteries hardened quicker than usual. A heart transplant could certainly be a gift of many extra years of healthy life, but it was not a certainty or a cure.

I knew Hannah might change her mind today but didn't think she would. She'd been distraught a few days earlier to still be in hospital for her twelfth birthday. But light had at last flickered in her eyes again when Andrew, Oli, Lucy, Phoebe and Andrew's parents had arrived to celebrate and Hannah had sat on her bed wearing a crown with the words 'Birthday Girl' spelled out in glittering pink stones, surrounded by the people she loved. She would soon return to them after three long months away.

'How do you think Hannah feels about a transplant?' I had been asked before the doctors left to go and see her.

'I'm almost sure she hasn't changed her mind. She knows what she wants.'

In some ways I didn't think Hannah was strong enough to cope with so many strangers asking her such an important question, and part of me didn't want them to. But I also knew the doctors had to be sure she wasn't being pressed into saying no to a transplant and I wanted them to understand that Hannah knew her own mind after so many years of ill health which was why I trusted her to make this decision. I had watched her strive to have a normal life, and seeing her do so had given me strength as well – to believe in her and fight for her if I needed to. Hannah had taught me to have the courage of my convictions and it was only now as it was tested beyond concrete reason into innate faith that I realised this.

As I sat in the room and waited, I thought about it all again. When Hannah was young and unable to tell me clearly what she wanted, I'd done what I thought was best for her. But now she knew for herself, and however closely I had walked by Hannah's side I had not walked in her shoes: she was the person who had lived with this for so long – and now could die with it too. If a transplant was too high a price for her to pay then I would accept that, however hard it was for me. Most importantly, I knew that I could not force her to have an operation she did not want or make her live on my terms. Hannah was not a small child any more, she was too old to cajole into doing something she didn't want, and she had shown me her determination again and again.

I knew that now, with the doctors in the room, she might reconsider and say yes to the transplant. But I would support her decision whatever it was. How did I have the courage to do this? Because I had seen both sides of the coin. I had been both a nurse and a mother of a sick child and knew a gulf divided the two. However many years a doctor spent training, however expert in their field and considered their professional opinion, they couldn't live a life that was another's. This was about Hannah. She was the only person who could ultimately decide what was right for her. And as I waited while the doctors went to speak to her, I knew that I would respect her choice – whatever it was.

CHAPTER NINE

Face Your Fears

❀

When I first started getting ill again, I got pains in my side as I lay in bed at night. But then Mum would take me to the doctors, they'd check me over and say I was fine. So we'd go home, I'd go to bed again and try lying on different sides to see if the pain was just a fluke. When it kept coming back I knew it wasn't, and that's when I ended up in Hereford Hospital with Dad where the pain got really bad. I can't remember much about it because I felt so tired but I know a nurse gave me an oxygen mask which I didn't like because I've never liked anything covering my face. I don't know why. I just hate it. Then I was put into an ambulance when all I wanted to do was sleep, and after I got to Birmingham a doctor started trying to stick needles into me. I cried and cried as I asked him to stop.

I felt really sad to be back in hospital – the same walls, the same doctors every day. They were all really nice but I wished things could be like they had been – me at school with Simone, bouncing around and just a few pills to take every day. That's why I didn't want the pacemaker at first when Mum told me about it. I wanted to be the same old me. But in the end I said OK because my heart couldn't pump properly without the Dobutamine and I needed something else to help it. So I agreed to have the operation and hoped that would be the end of everything. Mum told me the pacemaker caused no end of problems for poor Dr de Giovanni, though. She said he came out of the first operation in a real sweat and had to use special glue to stick my skin together.

I couldn't believe it when the wires didn't fit my heart first time. Who else would that happen to? It felt as if nothing ever went right for me. Doctors always say they won't hurt you and they'll do things differently to the time before. But I don't always believe them because once you've been in pain you don't know what to think, and after I had the pacemaker finished off I just wanted to go home.

That's when the doctors from Great Ormond Street came to see me about a transplant and I knew things were really serious. Mum had told me that I might need a new heart and I remember crying about it because I'd expected to get fixed and go home again. But I wasn't prepared for something as big as a transplant and knew it must be really bad when the doctors from Great Ormond Street came to see me in Birmingham because they don't go that far for someone who's well. They talked to me for ages and I understood what they were saying. I've had to think about my body all my life and knew they meant that I wouldn't get better without a transplant. But I didn't want to see any more doctors or have anyone else looking in on my life. I'd had enough of that.

Dad was in the room with me when the doctors showed me pictures of children who'd had successful transplants and got well again. But they also told me there was a risk that my body could reject the heart and I'd need to take medicines for ever to stop that happening because I'd be in trouble if it did. So it seemed to me that there were good and bad bits about a transplant but I knew what I wanted. I'd listened to the doctors carefully but was sure a transplant wasn't for me: it involved too many risks and I might be worse off than before. I didn't want that to happen but most of all I wanted to be at home, not lying in a hospital bed. I'd spent long enough in one of those and wanted to be somewhere I could smell fresh air and see the sun, hear Oli, Lucy and Phoebe playing and see Mum and Dad. I didn't want to be stuck in hospital even longer having an operation that might not even work. I wasn't willing to take that chance and I wanted to live my life. So I told the doctors what I wanted.

I guess they were a bit shocked and I don't know what other children might have felt. They might not have decided what I did. But I thought of the drains, the medicines and the biopsies and knew that I'd rather go home than have all of those again. I just wanted to enjoy my life. I wanted to be where I was happy even though I knew what it meant to say no to the transplant. I understood that I might die.

But it was hard choosing because you don't expect to have to think about something as big as a transplant at my age and I was scared because I didn't know what would happen if I said no – whether I'd be told off or forced into having it. But I didn't want anyone interfering in my decision or for Mum and Dad to make it for me. I knew they could if I wanted them to, but what would happen if it turned out wrong and they felt guilty if I died? I didn't want that to happen.

I've realised since that lots of mums and dads wouldn't have let their children make that kind of decision. Most parents would choose for their children who'd be happy to go along with what their mum and dad said. Some go all around the world looking for cures, and if they find one that's good. But some end up coming back seriously ill and die because the trip took a toll on them. That's a waste of what could have been the last month of their life at home or in hospital or seeing their family.

Have you read *The Witches* by Roald Dahl? It's about a boy who gets turned into a mouse when he accidentally stumbles in on a witches' convention. But his grandmother helps him to get rid of them because she trusts him when he comes up with a plan about how to do it, which means the children are safe from the horrible hags who'd turn them into mice.

My mum and dad trusted me as well, and I sometimes think adults should do it more. Some of them think children aren't old enough to understand things, and I know some aren't if they tell lies or don't think about things properly. But good children should be listened to and believed. It's about respecting them because there are some parents who don't – like the ones who don't feed or wash their children, or split up, get back together, split up again and forget that the children are in the middle of it all. There are lots of little ways some parents don't respect their children, and one of them is not listening when they have something to say or thinking that just because a child hasn't lived a lot of years they don't know anything. I know that's not true.

It's not up to me to say that all children should choose for themselves like I did because they might not want to – they might want their parents to do it for them. But I wanted to choose and I'm glad my mum and dad let me. You've got to have trust, otherwise you wouldn't get anywhere. I've had to trust the doctors to look after me, and since my heart has got bad I've had to trust my body to get rid of a cold or something if I give it time. It gives me strength when I trust myself and know my body will get its energy back.

I'm glad my mum trusts me too because if she didn't then I'd feel very small, like I wasn't important. Another reason I wanted to choose was because I think that if we all relied on our parents too much then we wouldn't get anywhere or learn anything. I realised that when I was at school and brought home my school diary at the end of the week for Mum to sign. I chucked it on the desk and expected her to do it, but she didn't, so when I got to school on Monday I realised it hadn't been done. But as I thought about it I knew that Mum doesn't forget things easily – she was just busy – and I should have taken responsibility to get the diary signed.

So I'm glad she trusted me when I really needed her to and I'm happy she and Dad let me decide for myself. If people don't like it, they can lump it, and I didn't say no to the transplant because I was scared. I thought about everything and decided. I'm not going to give up without a fight.

When the doctors had gone, I opened the door to Hannah's room and walked inside. Dwarfed by the machines around her, she was pale, almost grey, as she looked at me.

'What did they say, Han?' I asked as I sat down beside her.

'They talked to me about a transplant,' she said, her voice quiet but steady. 'They asked if I would like one.'

She was silent for a moment before starting to talk again.

'They say I'm very sick and might die or my life might be shorter if I don't have the transplant. But transplants don't last for ever, and if I have this one I might have to have another one in the future.'

Her gaze was firm as she looked at me.

'I don't want to take a heart that someone else wants more than me. It's better they give it to a child who really wants it, isn't it, Mummy?'

I couldn't speak as she looked at me.

'They said I could meet someone who'd had a transplant,' Hannah said.

'Do you want to?' I whispered.

'No. I'm not going to change my mind. I'm tired of being in hospital all the time. I want to go home.'

'You know you might die if you don't have the transplant, don't you, my darling?' I said softly.

'But I might die if I have it.'

I took her hand as I spoke again.

'I want you to know that Mummy and Daddy support your decision, but if you ever decide that you want us to choose for you or change your mind then we'll take you straight down to Great Ormond Street. You must always remember that.'

'I won't. The doctors don't know everything, Mummy. I proved them wrong when I was little, and I'll do it again. I'll get better.'

It was then I realised for the first time that a heart can break even as it is filling with hope.

The page was livid red as I stared at it, the colour of danger. It was a document formalising Hannah's decision, and its bright red urgency was an immediately identifiable signal to anyone looking at her medical notes. The Do Not Resuscitate order was a legally binding instruction which explained that if Hannah's heart failed she was not to be artificially resuscitated. There would be no ventilators, defibrillators or respirators. She would be allowed to die naturally if her heart gave up its fight. Hannah's decision to say no to a transplant had signalled to everyone involved in her care that she was prepared to die. She knew it was a possibility, and now, if the worst happened, no one would fight to bring her back.

Even though I had always known this was the ultimate consequence of Hannah's decision, a gulf can separate what we know to be true and what our hearts still resist. Even as the wheels had ground into motion for giving Hannah palliative care at home – the kind given to relieve symptoms rather than cure a life-threatening illness – I'd resisted thinking about her possible death. And as she was assigned a social

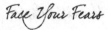

worker to liaise with home support services and given a place at Acorns Children's Hospice in Worcester, I'd told myself that Hannah's life was limited, just as I'd always known it might be after she was diagnosed with cardiomyopathy, but her illness was not definitely terminal. No one knew what the future held.

But when I met with Dr Wright a few days before we left hospital, I knew I had to ask the question I'd been putting off for so long. Until then an irrational voice inside had stopped me speaking my fears – as if talking about them would betray Hannah by allowing the creeping poison of doubt to erode my hope – but I knew I had to.

'How long do you think she has?' I asked Dr Wright as we sat together.

He looked at me steadily. We had never spoken about this. The medics had taken their lead from Andrew and me and not provided answers to questions we hadn't asked.

'I can't say for sure, Mrs Jones,' he replied.

'But do you have any idea?'

'Nothing is certain, but if I had to I would say Hannah has three months, possibly six.'

Guilt had rushed through me. What kind of mother was I to even ask such a question? Hannah needed me to be hopeful, didn't she? My tears ran slowly at first, coming thicker and faster as I shook, physically shocked at hearing out loud what I almost knew, and an even greater urgency to take Hannah home filled me. This was an opinion, not a certainty, as Dr Wright himself had told me, and the only thing I could be sure of is that I would help Hannah to live as she wanted, make sure she was happy while I hoped for a miracle. Other people might think we were going home to die, but I knew that we were not. Hannah wanted to live and my questions could not hasten her death, just as they could not make her survive. Hope could sustain both of us though.

Such feelings of acceptance and denial would be the paradox that I lived every day from now on: knowing Hannah could die but hoping she would get stronger. What gave me the strength to sustain this tussle between realism and hope? Hannah. She had taught me how to live in a different way – to have the courage of my convictions, seize the day and embrace it. She had made a choice and now I would live it with her. Hannah was so much more than her illness. We would let each day unfold one by one as we gleaned as much pleasure as possible from them.

I knew that Hannah, like me, understood the implications of what was happening. After the Great Ormond Street team had come to see her, I'd talked to her again about her decision. But while I wanted her to understand what it meant, I didn't want her to be afraid of death, counting down time instead of enjoying it. So when she giggled about what the doctors had said, I'd joined in her laughter. I wanted her to be positive because if she didn't have that then there was little else for us to cling onto. Everything concrete was stacked against Hannah – the results of her heart scans, the doctors' expectations and her complicated drug regime. But life isn't just about what we can see, measure and touch, it is about how we feel, and being positive would not only help Hannah to enjoy her life, but maybe prolong it.

'They don't know it all, do they, Mum?' she'd say. 'I'll get better when I go home, won't I?'

'I hope so, darling.'

'The doctors think I might die, but they don't know, do they?'

'Not always, Han. We need to let your pacemaker settle so we're going home to enjoy ourselves and we'll see what happens.'

The only concern Hannah expressed was that I would not be able to cope with her at home because her care was still very intensive – in addition to the complexity of the Dobutamine line, there were about ten other drugs that she would need every day, oxygen tanks and a nasogastric tube to help with her feeding.

'I don't want to make you work too hard,' she would tell me.

'I won't. I will have lots of help, we can go to Acorns for a rest, and we'll be fine. I don't want you to worry that looking after you is too difficult for me. It never will be.'

A few days later we left hospital and arrived at Acorns Hospice on the outskirts of Worcester where we were going to stay for two weeks as a transition from hospital to home. I felt overwhelmed as Hannah was stretchered inside and I walked beside her into the 'hub' area at the building's heart. It was a light room with windows along one side which opened into the garden. Shelves lined with films and books filled one wall and there were huge sofas covered in cushions. It was a home from home, and after so long in hospital I could hardly believe we were here – the first step to making Hannah's dream a reality.

Running off the hub were the kitchen and dining area, an art room and more windows overlooking a play area. Two corridors also led to the hospice's bedrooms, and the whole building was full of light and colour. But it was perhaps in Hannah's bedroom that the thoughtfulness of the care at Acorns was most obvious. The soft duvet had been made up with a pink cover, just as the staff knew she liked, and a lavender bag hand embroidered with the letter 'H' was lying on her pillow. Pink roses stood in a jar on the bedside table, and a door opened onto the garden. Through large windows Hannah could see the sun shining, grass, flowers and sky, and as she was put into bed a shard of the worry which had made her face drawn for so long began to fade.

'It's beautiful, Mummy,' she said as she looked around. 'Oli, Lucy and Phoebe can visit me now. When are they coming?'

'Tomorrow, I think. Daddy too.'

'I can't wait to see them.'

Over the next few days we settled in at Acorns, and the help and support offered by everyone there soothed both Hannah and me. After months spent in hospital, little things meant a great deal – soft carpet beneath our feet, newly washed clothes, doors wide enough to let wheelchairs pass easily through, and fresh food served by the half spoonful to tempt a sick child. Most important of all, though, was being in a place surrounded by people who either had a sick child or were expert in dealing with life-limiting conditions. Our hospice coordinator, Julia, was a particular support because I felt she understood why Hannah had decided as she had done – and why Andrew and I had let her. It was a great comfort to me.

We had been due to stay at Acorns for two weeks but ended up staying a month after floods made roads impassable and shut down electricity supplies. Hannah was content to be there but still wanted to make the final journey back home to the place she knew, with the people she loved. So as the time drew near for us to leave Acorns, I drove home one day to get Hannah's room ready before stopping off for petrol on the way back to the hospice.

'What do you think you're doing?' a man shouted, as I got out of the car in a daze. 'You've come in the wrong way. You've jumped the queue.'

'I'm sorry,' I said. 'I didn't realise.'

'Well, that's no use to me, is it?'

'I'm sorry,' I said again.

'So just move your car.'

I looked at him blankly, unable to understand how someone could get so angry about something so small. But I said nothing as the man let his anger stream out of him and people watched. I didn't want to argue. I knew more than ever now that some battles weren't worth fighting. But there were some I would do anything to win.

I could see their faces as we turned into the drive. Andrew, Oli, Lucy and Phoebe were watching at a window for us, waiting for us to come home, and the children ran outside as I pulled up the car.

'Mummy!' Phoebe cried, and I lifted her into my arms. 'Where have you been? Grandma has bought me a whole bag of clothes and I want to show you.'

She carried on chatting, a stream of words tumbling out of her mouth, as Lucy pulled open Hannah's door.

'You're here!' she exclaimed. 'We've got a new DVD, and Dad has got pizza.'

Hannah smiled as her sisters chatted and Oli stood quietly in the background, trying to get a word in edgeways but unable to find a gap in the girls' excitement.

'Welcome home,' Andrew said with a smile as I put Phoebe down and went to open the boot of the car to get Hannah's wheelchair. 'Why don't I carry her?'

Andrew reached into the car to put his arms around Hannah and she blinked in the sunlight as he lifted her out.

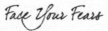

She looked pale and slight in her father's arms, a ghost of the girl who'd burst in from school and shared out her sweets. The Dobutamine line peeped out of her jumper and a naso-gastric tube ran under her nose. Reaching into the car, I took out her syringe driver and followed Andrew as he started carrying Hannah inside

'We've done lots to your room,' Lucy cried as she followed. 'We've made pictures, and got you flowers too.'

The children crowded behind us as Andrew carried Hannah upstairs to her room. Pointing out the welcome banners they'd made and the pictures they'd painted for their sister, they talked excitedly as Andrew sat Hannah down on the edge of the bed and she looked around.

'My room smells nice,' she said and smiled.

Her hands flitted up to her face, curling around her nose and mouth. It was a gesture Hannah made whenever she was happy or excited, and I hadn't seen her do it for so long. She was happy. She was home.

Lucy sat beside Hannah as she lay on her bed stroking Tails McFluff. The sun was shining outside and I'd just opened her bedroom window to let the smell of early autumn into the room. It hung in the air – a hint of wood smoke and the promise of slight dampness later – but for now the soft breeze brought sunshine with it as it drifted in. I'd just changed Hannah's bed sheets and brought a pair of warm pyjamas up from the kitchen where I'd ironed them. Lucy was chatting to Hannah as I left them to go downstairs again.

'Did I tell you what Mr Minty did yesterday?' I could hear her say. 'He tried to buck me off after clearing a three-foot jump, but I didn't let him!'

The girls giggled and I smiled to myself.

This was how Hannah had spent most of her time since coming home from Acorns. Still very weak, she struggled with the side effects of the powerful drugs she was taking and often had bad diarrhoea or sickness. The medication also affected her eyesight so she couldn't read and got very bad headaches that made her lie quietly as she waited for the pain to ease.

But, even so, Hannah was part of our family life again: she could hear the door bang when Lucy went out to ride her pony, a shout of triumph as Oli won his computer game or Phoebe's cries as she played. The girls in particular were also very conscious to make sure they brought the outside in to Hannah. So Lucy came home from riding with brightly coloured leaves or a handful of blackberries that she'd picked, while Phoebe literally dug her heels in to get fresh flowers for her sister.

'Stop!' she'd shouted one day as she left the house for school. 'Look!'

She was pointing to two tiny crocuses which had flowered overnight on the lawn. We were running late and a taxi was waiting to take her to school because I couldn't leave Hannah.

'She won't be long,' I said to the driver and watched Phoebe pick the flowers before going inside, putting them in an egg cup and walking upstairs.

'Look what God grew for you last night,' she said to Hannah, who smiled when she saw the purple splashes that spoke of a new season.

It was moments like this that made Hannah happy, just as stroking the cat or eating a morsel of food she particularly liked did, and it comforted me to know that pleasure found in the tiniest moments can make a life worth living.

Our days were completely unpredictable. On good ones, Hannah could get out of bed and bump downstairs on her bottom while I carried the heavy syringe driver containing her Dobutamine so that she could watch some television in the lounge or just sit with us. Within a couple of months of coming home she'd also started going to the local hospital school for a few hours on the morning of days when she felt well enough. So after disconnecting her central line I would put her into a taxi for the fifteen-minute journey to hospital, where a nurse would reconnect her as soon as she arrived.

Otherwise our routine was very like it had been when Hannah came home following the chemotherapy because I was with her constantly – never far in case of a problem with the Dobutamine line, giving her medication every two hours from 7 a.m. to 10 p.m. and checking on her throughout the night. District nurses visited every day for half an hour, but they could only do observations or check up on Hannah rather than practically care for her because they could not attend to her Dobutamine line. So other than the hours when she was at hospital school, it would be three months before I could leave Hannah in someone else's care. When nurses trained to look after the Dobutamine started making a four-hour round trip from Bristol three times a week, I was finally able to do the school run, catch up on washing and look after the thousand tiny details of caring for everyone.

Once again, looking after my well children and a very sick one was more of a juggling act than a properly executed plan. Oli, Lucy and Phoebe quickly learned that on bad days, when Hannah was poorly, my attention was focused solely on her and we all switched into 'sick' mode – Phoebe sitting almost quietly in front of the television, Lucy getting her sister ready for bed or preparing her some simple food and Oli helping out as well. On a day when Hannah was barely conscious, he had helped me carry her to the bathroom where he'd sat with her as she lay in the water, quietly keeping watch over his big sister, while I went to change her bed sheets. Just ten years old, his quiet kindness humbled me.

There were many times when I wanted to split myself in two so that I could look after everyone. But if Hannah was short of breath or in pain, I couldn't leave her to even run to the loo or kiss Phoebe good night. My physical presence was the only thing which reassured her, and each storm she weathered frightened me. As her condition dipped, I would give her as many of the drugs I was able to, like diuretics or morphine, to try and control her symptoms before calling our GP or the hospital for help if I couldn't. Some nights felt like for ever as I sat with her and waited to see if her body would win its fight, or whether it would lose it, and these were the only moments when Hannah became scared.

'I'm frightened, Mummy,' she would moan breathlessly as her hands reached out for me.

On nights like those the question of a transplant would press into the front of my thoughts again, and I would talk to Hannah about it when she had recovered a little.

'You know you can always change your mind about the transplant, don't you, Han?' I would ask. 'And if you decide that you want it then I can let the doctors know.'

'I don't,' she would tell me before turning over, signalling to me that she didn't want to talk about it any more.

I wasn't the only one who asked her. Many of the professionals we came into contact with – doctors, specialists, nurses, carers and a social worker – questioned Hannah about the transplant, and I understood why. But it also frustrated me because I wanted Hannah's choice to be respected, not doubted. I wished people could accept it because the questions were obviously too much for her at times.

'I don't want to talk about it any more,' she would tell me. 'Why does everyone keep asking?'

'Because they want to be sure that you know you can change your mind.'

'But I do.'

She even nicknamed one nurse The Wicked Witch of the West because she seemed so unable to understand what Hannah had decided, and I had to laugh when she did.

'I want everyone to leave me alone,' Hannah would say. 'I want them to stop asking.'

But after a particularly bad night or day, Hannah would start to stabilise and I would breathe a sigh of deep relief as our life slipped back into the pattern we had created for it. We all lived a rollercoaster existence, but Oli, Lucy and Phoebe's ability to accept it taught me more forcefully than ever before about just how adaptable children can be – up one day and down the next.

I learned to live that with them as they became 'ordinary' children again – fighting over the last biscuits in the tin or asking if I would help them with homework – and Hannah watched some television, played a game of cards or tried to

read. When the children were at school I would do house-
hold jobs before going to sit in her room to brush her hair or
read stories until everyone else came home and Oli, Lucy or
Phoebe tumbled into her room to chat. On the Sundays when
Hannah felt well, Andrew took us all to the pub which was an
outing she particularly loved.

We were all pleased to be together again, and each of my
children told me how they felt in their different ways: Oli, by
sitting a little closer as we watched TV and Phoebe, by hanging onto me for a moment longer than necessary as we
cuddled. But as ever, it was Lucy who was the most outspoken
one about how she felt after I found her huddled under her
duvet reading by torchlight.

'What are you up to?'

'I can't stop reading because this story is too exciting.'

'Well, I think you might have to. It's late, Lucy. You need
to sleep.'

She put the book down beside her bed and stretched up
her arms towards me.

'Can I have a biscuit, please?' she asked as she grinned
hopefully.

'Just this once then.'

'Thanks, Mum.'

Lucy leaped out of bed to rush to the kitchen before
suddenly stopping.

'It's lovely to have you home,' she said. 'I missed you and
Hannah when you weren't here.'

I was sitting outside with my friend Lindy beside me. It was about 1 a.m. and the sky was black above us. Although it was cold, we'd been sitting out here ever since I'd finally got Hannah to sleep. Lindy had understood when I'd called to ask her to come over and had waited for me to come downstairs before handing me a mug of tea.

'Did I tell you who I saw at the horse sales?' she said, and slipped into a stream of chatter as I sipped.

This was what Lindy always gave me – a comforting glimpse of the everyday world which I needed to hear after a particularly dark day. She told me about the village, school and any bits of gossip she'd heard as I sat with my thoughts. Lindy had lost her husband and knew what it was like to grieve – the aching emptiness, the physical feeling of heaviness which filled me on days when Hannah was at her weakest and I knew how close we were to the edge of the unknown.

In the rush of the emergency I could lose myself in constant practical tasks – medication and comfort, calling doctors for advice or waiting for them to arrive. But when Hannah was finally stable again and asleep, my fears crept out of the darkest corners of my mind and questions filled the silence. Those were the times when I cried as I sat outside and stared up at a dark sky, trying to make sense of it all.

There were moments now when I was more afraid than I ever had been, and I felt very alone after leaving the safety of the hospital because although there were always doctors and nurses on the end of the phone, they weren't physically with me. I was the one who sat with Hannah and gave her pain relief or turned on her oxygen to help ease her breathing when her skin went grey. Andrew was often away with work during the week, which meant I was alone, and although I knew I could call him any time it was hard to know when to draw the line and phone to say that Hannah was dangerously ill. Was it when she moaned in fear or when I had to give her a second dose of medication? It happened frequently, and I couldn't call Andrew every time. He was working hard to support us all and I knew his constant efforts on behalf of his family outside the home were just as important as mine within it. I phoned him when I needed to talk and had asked him to come home a couple of times, which he did without question, wherever he was in the country.

But when Andrew was away I almost dreaded the quiet hours when Hannah had finally fallen asleep and the house was quiet. So I would call Lindy and we would sit together – sometimes talking about small, everyday things, at others quietly discussing some of my doubts and fears which clamoured most loudly. Was Hannah comfortable enough? Were Oli, Lucy and Phobe all right? Was I doing the best I could for all of them? Were Hannah's medications right? Was she becoming withdrawn? Was she afraid?

Hannah never spoke about her fears, but I knew what they were because I shared them. Being told that your child might die is something that takes just a few seconds; accepting it is a process which never ends. I could feel doubt and hope constantly intertwine inside me, and if I thought about losing Hannah a raw fear would make me almost physically ache. If I had to think about it because she was particularly ill, I would lose myself in practicalities. I'd seen death many times as a nurse and knew it did not have to be painful. But could it ever be that simple? The thing that scared me most was the thought of Hannah suffering, and I knew I would do anything to soothe her. I wanted her to feel peaceful and unafraid whatever happened.

'Dying is like going to sleep,' I told her one night, just as I had done when she was small and asked about it. 'It doesn't hurt. I'll be with you. I'll always be here.'

We didn't speak about it again, and Hannah was always keen to forget when she recovered. But it frightened me each time she deteriorated and I wondered if I could bear the weight of being completely responsible if the worst happened. I was afraid that I wouldn't be strong enough for her.

Sometimes, as I tried to calm my thoughts, I read a poem I'd been given by a nurse at Acorns. She had given it to me in an envelope and told me to look at it when I felt ready. But when I'd opened up the envelope and read what was on the piece of paper inside, it had spoken to me. I knew I had to have faith if I was going to do my best for Hannah.

Now I handed the poem to Lindy, who took it, leaning towards the porch light to read. She didn't have to say the words aloud as she did. I knew the poem off by heart.

> I'll lend you, for a little while,
> A child of mine, God said.
> For you to love the while he lives,
> And mourn for when he's dead.
> It may be six or seven years
> Or forty-two or three.
> But will you, till I call him back,
> Take care of him for Me?
>
> He'll bring his charms to gladden you
> And, should his stay be brief,
> You'll have his lovely memories
> As solace for his grief.
> I cannot promise he will stay,
> Since all from earth return,
> But there are lessons taught below,
> I want this child to learn.

I've looked the whole world over,
In my search for teachers true,
And from the folk that crowd life's lane
I have chosen you.
Now will you give him all your love,
And not think the labour vain?
Nor hate me when I come to take
This lent child back again?

I fancied that I heard them say,
'Dear Lord Thy Will Be Done'
For all the joys thy child will bring
The risk of grief we'll run.
We'll shower him with tenderness,
We'll love him while we may,
And for the happiness we've known
Forever grateful stay.

But should the angels call for him
Much sooner than we planned,
We'll bear the bitter grief that comes
And try to understand.

Lindy didn't speak as she slipped her hand over mine. She would wait until I felt ready to talk. For now we would sit together. Just like Hannah, it comforted me to have someone close by.

The room was completely still as I sat beside Hannah. She was lying unconscious and I was waiting to see if she would stir, watching her face, wondering if now was the day, hour or minute when I would lose her. Three days ago she had suddenly and severely deteriorated, and I'd phoned the doctor in the middle of the night. Hannah had been put onto morphine, but even with it she was still distressed and I'd asked if she wanted to go to Acorns.

'Yes, Mummy,' she'd replied, her face drawn with pain. 'I'm very tired now.'

An ambulance had brought us here, and within hours Hannah had fallen unconscious. I'd stayed with her ever since – only leaving to snatch some sleep, knowing that a nurse would come and get me if I was needed. The days had blurred one into another, hours slipping by in the silence of the room as I talked to Hannah, telling her about what we were going to do at Christmas, which was just a few days away. She'd been looking forward to it, and the presents she'd asked me to buy for every-one were hidden under her bed waiting to be wrapped.

'Will Hannah wake up soon, Mummy?' Phoebe had asked when Andrew, Oli, Lucy and Phoebe had arrived to see us earlier that day.

'I don't know, darling,' I replied, and the brightness of Phoebe's chatter had filled the silent air.

They had all just left the room to go to the Acorns carol service and I stood up as I heard the music start. Walking down the corridor, I went into the hub and stood beside them as the first carol was sung and Phoebe slipped her hand into mine. It felt warm, solid, and I thought of Hannah lying so quietly.

'Are there any children too sick to be here today?' a woman who had played the harp asked as the concert came to an end.

'My sister is asleep in her room,' Lucy told her. 'I think she'd like to hear a carol. She likes music very much.'

'And what's your sister's name?' the woman asked gently.

'Hannah.'

'That's a pretty name. Do you know what carol she would like?'

Lucy thought for a moment.

'Little Town of Bethlehem.'

Lucy wanted to play with the harpist, so Andrew and I walked with her to Hannah's room where we stood around the bed.

'Do you think Hannah will like it, Mummy?' Lucy asked.

'I'm sure she will,' Andrew replied, knowing that I could not speak.

Soon the sound of the music filled the room, and I felt sure Hannah could hear it. I thought of the notes, weaving their way into the darkest recesses of her mind as she lay unconscious. Would they tell her that Christmas was nearly here?

I will never know if Hannah heard the music or not, but within twenty-four hours she started moving a little and scratching her skin. It was clear she was beginning to move out of deep unconsciousness into a place where she could feel the effects of the morphine, and over the next day she gradually woke up as her pain relief was reduced. Like a butterfly slowly emerging from its cocoon, Hannah came back to us.

'Is it Christmas yet?' she asked drowsily when she could finally speak.

'No. Not yet.'

'My presents.'

I thought of them lying in shopping bags underneath her bed.

'They're waiting for you, Han. They're still where you left them.'

'I need to wrap them,' she said, her voice weak but audible.

Late on Christmas Eve, we arrived home to find that Andrew, Oli, Lucy and Phoebe had decorated a tiny tree for Hannah which stood in the corner of her bedroom. They had also strung fairy lights up around her window which shone as she was propped up on pillows in bed the next morning while Oli, Lucy and Phoebe opened the presents she'd given them.

'Thanks, Hannah,' Oli said as he looked at his Nintendo game. 'Shall we do yours for you?'

'I want to open one too!' Phobe cried.

'After me,' her brother said.

'And me!' Lucy insisted.

They all started ripping paper as Hannah watched and a weak smile stole across her face. Later that day she got out of bed for long enough to join us at Christmas lunch, unable to eat but wanting to be part of the day. I hurriedly had my food before carrying her into the sitting room where we sat together. Drops of coloured light shone on the Christmas tree and bounced off the tinsel strewn all over it. I could hear Oli, Phoebe and Lucy laughing with Andrew at the table and the television burbling softly as Hannah watched it. All I could do was wonder at the strength of spirit which had brought her home to us. Hannah's determination to carry on living had willed her back from the very edges of life.

The phone rang as darkness fell on a Friday afternoon in late January 2008. The day before I'd taken Hannah into Hereford Hospital where she'd had an echocardiogram to check her progress after coming off the Dobutamine. She'd wanted to stop taking it because the heavy syringe driver feeding the drug into her bloodstream made it impossible to do something as simple as go downstairs to get a drink or reach up to get a book from a shelf. Hannah was dependent on me or someone else for help, and felt like a prisoner.

It wasn't the life that she'd wanted when she'd decided to come home. Hannah didn't like being trapped here any more than she did in hospital. We'd always known the Dobutamine wasn't a long-term treatment for her heart failure, and it was six months now since she'd left hospital. So at a meeting attended by doctors, nurses and social workers involved in her care it was agreed to let Hannah come off the drug, and a few days ago I'd taken her into hospital where the Dobutamine had been slowly reduced as her vital statistics were monitored.

It was an anxious twenty-four hours, but Hannah's pulse had stayed exactly where it was, her breathing was easy and she was pain free. It was now a question of taking it day by day, and although no one knew exactly how Hannah was coping without the Dobutamine – whether the pacemaker had strengthened her heart muscles or her body had just learned to function with such low cardiac function – it was clear that she was.

But yesterday we'd seen a locum doctor we didn't know well for a follow-up scan and I had felt uneasy when the question had been raised about whether she wanted to go back onto the Dobutamine. Alarm bells immediately started ringing because Hannah had only just come off the drug and I didn't understand why this doctor was asking about it again, so I'd confronted him angrily after she had left the room.

'This has only just been decided,' I told him. 'I don't understand why you are questioning her.'

We had left quickly and I had gone home simmering that this doctor seemed unable to accept a decision so many people had agreed. But we were having Oli's birthday party at the weekend and there was a lot to do, so by the next day I'd almost forgotten the locum doctor as I walked to pick up the phone when it rang.

'Mrs Jones?' a voice said.

'Yes.'

'I'm sorry to call late but the doctor you saw yesterday has some concerns about Hannah.'

'What do you mean? She's here with me and she's fine.'

'He'd like to see her again.'

'But we came in yesterday. It's late, it's cold. I don't want to make her go out again.'

'So you don't want to bring Hannah back in?'

'No. I don't. She's fine. We can come in next week if you need us to.'

As the phone call ended I thought back to yesterday's meeting. I didn't understand why this doctor wanted to see Hannah again now, late on a Friday afternoon, but if he was going to ask her more questions about the Dobutamine then I wasn't going to take her in.

Soon Andrew arrived home and we started chatting about our plans for the weekend. Hannah was not up to much but the thought of Oli's birthday party was exciting for everyone.

'Can we have trifle, Daddy?' she asked Andrew as he got himself a cup of tea.

The children settled down to watch some television with Andrew while I did jobs in the kitchen, and it must have been about 5 p.m. when the phone rang again. I wondered who it was as I walked into the living room to see the colour draining from Andrew's face as he spoke. His voice was low as he repeatedly insisted that everything was fine.

'No,' he kept saying again and again. 'She's here. We're fine.'

I knew something was very wrong as I asked the children to go to their bedrooms and Andrew put down the phone.

'It was the hospital,' he said. 'They want us to take Hannah back in to start the Dobutamine again.'

Coldness spread through me.

'What?'

'They say that if we don't agree they're thinking of applying for a court order to make sure Hannah is treated. They said she could be forcibly removed from our care.'

'What do you mean?' I cried.

'They say they won't do anything until they know what we think. But we've got to tell them if we're prepared to take Hannah back to hospital.'

For a moment I felt almost dazed. A court order? Legal action? How could this be happening? Hannah was here with us, she was doing well without the Dobutamine. How could people talk about Hannah's choice and now try to foist another on her? Why were they doing this? Then my hands shook as adrenalin rushed through me: if the hospital authorities were considering court action to restart the Dobutamine, would they do the same about a transplant?

'I don't understand,' I said as Andrew and I looked at each other.

'Neither do I,' he replied.

'They can't threaten us.'

'I think they are.'

I had to think quickly, stem the panic inside me and decide what to do.

'Hannah doesn't want to be in hospital. She doesn't want the Dobutamine.'

'I know.'

'Then that's what we'll tell them.'

Andrew looked at me and I saw fear in his eyes about whether we could stop the juggernaut that was speeding towards us.

'We need a lawyer,' he said.

Both of us were quiet as we sat down and started searching through phone books. I didn't know how the courts worked, I'd never even spoken to a solicitor other than to buy a house, but knew the legal system could take our child from us. We had to stop this and needed to find someone to help us. But late on a Friday evening answer phones clicked on at the end of every number we tried.

I tried to stem the fear building inside me. Why was the hospital doing this? How could they think this was in Hannah's best interests? Everyone knew what she wanted. It had only just been agreed that she would stop having the Dobutamine.

'Can you help us?' I asked desperately when someone finally answered one of the solicitors' numbers I was trying.

'Everyone has gone home for the weekend,' the voice said coldly. 'Can you call back on Monday?'

I slammed down the phone and started pacing the room as I wondered who could help us and how we could stop this madness. The children knew something was wrong because my friend Tina had come over to look after them. But I wanted to stop this before it went any further and we had to tell them exactly what was happening.

The phone rang and I snatched the receiver.

'Kirsty?' a voice said.

It was a nurse we knew well and Hannah liked.

'A bed has been prepared for Hannah,' she told me and my hands started shaking. 'But if an ambulance is sent for her with the police, I've offered to come with it so at least Hannah will see a face she knows.'

I thought of blue lights flashing in the dark night, strangers coming to take my child, Hannah's face as she looked out of the window. How would she ever understand that we couldn't protect her from this? I could tell from the nurse's voice that she was distressed about what was happening, and her kindness stilled me for a moment at least. I thought of the hospital managers and lawyers talking over her head, locked in rooms discussing the case of a girl they didn't know. If the nurse understood how wrong this was then surely the hospital authorities would too? Wouldn't they realise and stop this from going any further? We had to convince them. But how?

Maybe I should have been afraid all along that something like this would happen, prepared myself for it because I had always known that there were those who couldn't understand Hannah's choice – and my support of it perhaps even more so. I'd looked into eyes over the past few months which had silently questioned me at best, accused me at worst. The doctors who knew Hannah well – like Dr Wright at Birmingham and Dr Meyrick at Hereford – had always respected our decisions. But on a few occasions I'd seen distrust deep in a person's gaze and had to steel myself against their doubts even as they touched the rawest nerve inside me. What kind of woman did these people see? A mother who wanted her child to die?

I understood that some people might not understand, how people who did not know us could wonder why I did not coax my child into having an operation that could give her years of good health. But a transplant was not a cure: Hannah knew what she wanted and I knew just as surely that I could never force her to have an operation she didn't agree to. Neither I, nor her doctors at Birmingham or Great Ormond Street, would countenance that.

But not everyone knew us as well as they did, and how to explain years of ill health and dashed hopes to virtual strangers who didn't know our story? How to encapsulate in neat conversation the experience of watching Hannah during all this time and understanding why she had had enough of hospital? How to describe the experience of learning that what she wanted was the most important thing? Not my grief, dreams or fears, but Hannah's wishes?

The hours passed in a blur until late in the evening when the hospital rang back. After talking to Great Ormond Street, who had explained how vital both Hannah's and our views were, the hospital had decided not to seek a court order that night. It comforted to me to know that Great Ormond Street was speaking reason, but I knew I had to agree when the hospital asked if a child protection nurse could come to see Hannah the next day before the matter was reconsidered by a barrister acting for the health authority on Monday morning.

I tried to calm myself as I wondered how we'd get through the next two days. We would focus on Oli's birthday and try to keep things as normal as possible. But even so I would have to tell Hannah that someone was coming to talk to her and how was I going to explain what was happening? How to make sense of the fact that, after fighting to bring her home, we might have to stop now? If a court ordered us to give Hannah up then we would be powerless to protect her, just as she needed us most.

Tomorrow a stranger would come into our house and sit down with Hannah before carrying our hopes – and fears – back to the people who were trying to rip our home apart. Our future lay in her hands.

CHAPTER TEN

Know Your Strength

❀

I didn't like the look of the doctor we went to see just before the hospital decided a court might have to take me away, and that never helps. You have to like someone to trust them, and he looked stern to me. Like a traffic warden who wants to stick a ticket on your car. So I went home thinking I didn't like him and I was right because that was when the hospital said they might make me go back. I was in my bedroom when Mum told me and I cried when I found out what was happening. I didn't understand why the hospital wanted to make me have the Dobutamine again, but when I asked Mum if she'd make sure they didn't she only said that she'd do her best. I knew it meant that she wasn't sure she'd be able to because when Mum knows she can do something she always says 'Yes'.

That's why I felt really nervous when the nurse came to talk to me. Mum, Dad, Grandma and Grandpa were all in the kitchen but it was just me in my room with the hospital woman for the talk. We sat in my bedroom for about an hour as she asked me questions and I found it hard to talk about it all again. But it was easy in another way because I can't always say all the things that are in my head if I'm with someone I know. I don't want someone I like or love to think I'm stupid or feel sad about what I say, so it was good that I didn't know the hospital woman because I could tell her everything I felt about the operation and anaesthetic, needles and drains. How boring it was in hospital, how much I just wanted to be left alone, how I wanted to be able to do what I wanted at home, why I didn't want to go back on the Dobutamine or have a transplant even though I knew I could die. I also told her that I didn't want Mum and Dad to decide for me and I was happy to be off the Dobutamine because the syringe driver was so heavy that I couldn't move anywhere. I told her everything.

It felt like she was in the room for ages, but when she left Mum came back in and told me how well I'd done because the woman had said I was 'remarkable'. It sounded good but Mum said we had to wait until a judge decided what was going to happen and it was horrible not knowing. I couldn't stop thinking about it, even though it was Oli's birthday and he opened his presents in my room and we had cake, which would usually be enough to get my mind off something.

This time it wasn't though, and I kept wondering whether the hospital was going to listen to what I had to say and believe it. But on Monday morning the woman rang and told Mum they weren't going to make me go back in. I was really happy and I knew Mum was too. The court was going to leave us alone and I was going to stay at home just like I wanted to. I was so happy that I cried.

Do you like Hercule Poirot? He makes me laugh how he's so stuck in his ways about things like his moustache and tie. But what's best about him is that when everyone else looks at the murder in the conventional way, he looks at it differently and gets the case solved. Poirot doesn't make rushed decisions. Instead he looks at everything carefully and weighs it all up, which is what I did with the transplant.

That's why I didn't understand why the hospital did not listen to me properly before scaring us. If anyone had tried to understand then they'd have known I didn't want to go back on the Dobutamine and surely you should ask someone's point of view properly before you get a judge and lawyers involved? I think the hospital could have taken a bit of advice from Hercule Poirot about considering all the facts.

It was a good thing I came off the Dobutamine because that was when I got stronger, and look at all the good things which happened after that: I met Prince Charles, had a holiday in Cornwall, went to the horse show with Lucy and was at home where I wanted to be doing the things I wanted to do. I think it's a lot for someone who's sick.

The weekend after the child protection nurse visited us was the longest of my life, and it felt almost unreal to watch Hannah sitting with Oli while he opened his birthday presents or settling her down to sleep at night knowing she might be taken from us. The idea that her trust in Andrew and me might be shattered was horrifying: we were the people who protected her, home was the place where she felt safe, and now it was under threat. I wondered if I could run, hide Hannah from the people who were threatening us, but knew it was impossible. All I could do was hope that the hospital official who'd spoken to her would see what others had – how considered and certain a twelve-year-old could be, how she understood that she might die without a transplant but wanted to be at home.

I knew that, for every person who'd doubted our decisions, there had been others brave enough to support them. But as the weekend dragged by I wondered again and again on which side the child protection nurse would be. If she believed in us then we would know once and for all that

Hannah's choice was going to be respected. If not, we would be hurled into court hearings and legal arguments.

It was about 11 a.m. on the Monday morning when the phone finally rang.

'Mrs Jones?'

My hands began to shake as I heard the child protection nurse's voice.

'Yes.'

'The hospital's legal advisers have met and a decision has been reached,' she said. 'They know that Hannah is very clear about not wanting to go back on the Dobutamine or have a transplant. She is sure of what she wants, and because of this no more legal action will be taken.'

I felt relieved at first, but then angry as Hannah cried when I told her the news. The hospital should never have started this, and when the child protection nurse came back to see us I asked for letters of apology to be written to the children because I did not want any of them to worry it might happen again in the future. But we had already been thrown back into everyday life by the time the letters arrived and so I tucked them away in a drawer, knowing they were there if I needed them in the future. There wasn't time to dwell on what had so nearly happened, and although I knew I'd never forget I made myself move on.

But the pointlessness of the hospital's actions had been proved every day since then because Hannah had got stronger after coming off the Dobutamine, slowly gaining stamina as the weeks passed, and starting to get out of bed on more days than she did not. I believed it was partly because she could move around more and also eat properly now that she was free of the Dobutamine syringe driver. Mostly, though, I was sure it was down to contentment as Hannah challenged herself to do more, and began to learn the new limits of her body after being so weak for so long. Like ancient sailors journeying to the edge of maps unsure of what they would find, Hannah tested her body bit by bit until it told her to stop. Then she would have to rest until she felt well enough to get out of bed again and see if she could push herself just a little more.

Her determination to do as much as possible never wavered and we learned to make the most of it when she felt a rush of energy. There was never any warning when it might come – Hannah could wake up feeling poorly and then rally at lunchtime, or she could have a whole day when she felt well. We just had to take the window of opportunity when it came, which meant we made more than one trip to the supermarket or to drop the children off at school in our pyjamas if Hannah suddenly felt well and we hadn't had time to change. There were often days when neither of us managed to get dressed by lunchtime if she was in bed resting and I was busy doing medications or chores. But if she told me she was feeling well and I knew we needed food then we would put on our coats and go shopping.

Sometimes Hannah could walk and on other days she needed her wheelchair, but she always insisted that I didn't use a trolley adapted for it.

'They're what old ladies use,' she would exclaim, and so I'd push her, a basket hanging off each of my arms and one on Hannah's lap for light things.

The first time we went out in our pyjamas, she worried that people would know what we were doing – the embarrassment of a typical almost teenager about doing something 'weird'. But when Hannah realised that no one had discovered our secret, she would giggle with me as we shopped. By late spring she was even able to go to Hereford occasionally, and on one warm day I parked the car in a disabled space close to the shops as we chatted.

'Where do you want to go?' I asked.

'I want new shoes,' Hannah replied. 'Simone has got some and I'd like some too.'

But as Hannah and I got out of the car I looked up to see a man glaring at us with his wife in the passenger seat beside him looking just as angry. I had obviously taken a space they wanted, and the two of them stared as I walked to open the boot and Hannah stood by the car. Now they looked even more annoyed. How dare I take a disabled space when my child and I were obviously well?

I pulled the wheelchair out of the car and unfolded it.

'Are you ready, Han?' I said and turned away from the stares.

It was something I'd had to learn to do, just as I had to smile when people exclaimed how well Hannah looked on days when there was pink in her cheeks. Her determination was a sometimes brilliant mask for her illness, and now as I pushed her towards town I could hear her breath catching. I didn't have to look at her face to know it would be pale with effort. By the time we got home she would have to go to bed to rest.

'How about we do this another day?' I asked.

'No!'

'I don't want you to get too tired, Han.'

'I won't.'

'Well, we'll go quick then, OK?'

'All right.'

It was the kind of quiet bargaining that Hannah and I had done again and again in recent months. Even as we tacitly acknowledged there would be a price to pay when she stretched herself, we didn't speak explicitly about it. Instead we quietly negotiated around the edges of Hannah's illness, and somehow she usually found the energy to do what she wanted before having to rest – sometimes for several days. I made sure she didn't take unnecessary risks but let her push herself, even though it scared me at times. But I couldn't let my fear create a new kind of prison for Hannah. I had to let her be. She would be thirteen soon and deserved some of the freedom that any other girl of her own age would enjoy. Anyway, as much as I wanted to fold her in my arms and keep her safe, Hannah wouldn't let me.

'So what kind of shoes do you want?' I asked as we neared the shop.

'I don't know. Something a bit girlie.'

I smiled. Hannah's school friends were beginning to abandon trainers in favour of more grown-up shoes and she wasn't going to be left behind.

❧

The horse lorry shuddered as it came to a stop and I jumped out.

'We've got to hurry!' I called to Lucy. 'We won't get you entered in all your classes if we don't do it soon.'

Lucy was being strangely slow today. Usually she was the one who could not wait to get to horse shows, but now she didn't seem to want to get out of the lorry.

'Will you catch me up?' I called as I got out and started walking towards the indoor school where the jumping competition was being held.

We were at a riding school about fifteen miles from our home and Lucy was going to compete with other local children. Andrew was at home with Hannah, Oli and Phoebe and was going to take them to the cinema. But as I walked I heard a stream of giggles behind me and turned to see Lucy walking to join me – with Hannah by her side.

'What are you doing here?' I asked. 'Did Daddy bring you?'

'No!' shrieked Hannah.

'What do you mean? How did you get here?'

'I hid!' she said triumphantly. 'Lucy helped me. I was in the bed right above your head!'

With peals of laughter, they explained how Lucy had helped Hannah hide under a duvet in the lorry's sleeping area which was why I'd been none the wiser

'Mum didn't know!' Lucy shrieked.

'She had no idea!' Hannah laughed.

I knew I should probably tell them off, but it was hard as they stood giggling with pleasure in front of me. For a moment I wondered what might happen if Hannah got short of breath because I didn't have any oxygen with me. But I didn't want to spoil the moment as I looked at her expectant face. I could stop her living her life because of my own fears.

'You won't send me home, will you?' Hannah asked, suddenly anxious as she realised that I might be angry. 'You won't phone Daddy?'

'Doesn't he know you're here?'

'No.'

'I think I'd better tell him, don't you?'

I rang home to let Andrew know where Hannah was and the girls looked at me hopefully as I finished the call.

'Hannah can stay,' I said, and they cheered. 'But you have to promise that you'll never stow away again. Daddy was really worried.'

'We promise,' they cried.

I was not completely surprised that Hannah had dared make this trip: she probably had four good days when she was up and about each week now and I was pretty sure that Lucy had also encouraged her. She was always cajoling Hannah into trying to do things, helping her forget her tiredness by making her laugh or shooing Phoebe out of the room on the days when Hannah was too tired to cope with her. Lucy was the one who pushed Hannah and bolstered her determination to do as much as possible because she, like Oli and Phoebe, had known nothing other than her sister's illness. It was a fact of life for the three of them which they accepted.

They knew it created limits, and when Hannah was ill I couldn't do things like take Lucy riding, drive Oli to football practice or read stories with Phoebe. But they did not see Hannah's condition as an obstacle, it was simply a part of our life, and that is why I will always remember the day at the horse show. Hannah was well, and for the first time in many months her illness completely receded into the background of our everyday life. Lucy entered her jumping classes and returned to us clutching rosettes while Hannah organised her – helping her fill out entry forms and sitting clutching a wooden spoon with a number on it to make sure the chips she ordered for them during breaks arrived safely.

'Isn't this great?' Hannah said as she turned to me late in the day. 'I want to come all the time from now on, Mum.'

Lucy started laughing as she looked at Hannah who, in her eagerness to eat her chips, had smeared her face with ketchup.

'You are so greedy!' Lucy exclaimed.

'You can talk,' Hannah cried.

As I looked at them I thought of the precious lesson I had learned with them during recent months: that focusing on the good in life, the here and now, can give you a strength you never knew was there. Children can quickly cast off unhappiness, and they had taught me to do the same. Just as Hannah refused to let her illness define her, I had learned to take the bad days in my stride before moving forward. And as I looked at Hannah and Lucy laughing I knew there was joy to be found in even the most ordinary moments – a streak of sunshine in a grey sky, the sound of laughter or the sight of a sister's face smeared with ketchup.

By late 2008 Hannah had started doing two mornings a week back at school. Too tired to manage it most of the time, she went in on the days when she felt strong enough, and her teachers at St Mary's did everything possible to help her – including reorganising Hannah's class timetable for the first three lessons of the day to make sure they were downstairs so she didn't have any steps to climb. She loved being part of school life again, however irregularly, and Simone would push her in a wheelchair from class to class as they chatted.

Other than school, Hannah had also started attending a weekly puppet group at the local church and going up to the stables to visit Lucy's horses whenever she could. She also continued to go to Acorns once a month, which had become a much-loved second home, and when she was well enough she helped me cook supper, groom the horses and even went to the dentist – something she hadn't done for years. Hannah's determination to live life to the full was proved every day.

It was more than a year now since she had left hospital, and Hannah had achieved the almost impossible – she was stronger, the pacemaker was doing its job well and although her heart function remained at just ten per cent, her body had somehow adapted. But while she was still adamant whenever the subject of the transplant was mentioned, no one could be sure when the spell that was keeping her strong might break. So when a charity offered us a once-in-a-lifetime opportunity, I knew we had to take it.

We applied for the trip with Caudwell Children after finding out about the charity from Acorns. They were taking forty children to Disney World Florida – a place we could never have visited without the paramedics, volunteers and doctors who would accompany the party – and at first I wasn't sure if Hannah was strong enough for such a long flight. But after talking to Dr Wright we decided that this was a unique opportunity for us as a family, and applied for places. The children were all as thrilled as each other when Caudwell Children accepted us, and their excitement just got more and more intense as the date approached.

But shortly before we were due to leave I got a phone call to say that Hannah was the only child out of forty going on the trip who had been refused insurance. Every company approached by Caudwell Children had told them she was too big a risk to cover, and if a new insurer could not be found then Hannah could not travel.

When the charity asked if they could issue a press release appealing for help, I agreed without a second thought. I just hoped that a small piece in a local paper might encourage someone to put up the surety the insurance company needed to cover Hannah, and an article soon appeared in a couple of local papers after the press release went out.

What I did not realise though is that the media is like a river which gathers momentum as it rushes down a hillside. After the first story appeared, we were contacted by a news agency who asked to do another and I agreed, thinking that the more coverage Hannah's plight got, the greater the chances of persuading someone to help with the insurance. As the journalist interviewed Hannah and me, we talked of all that had happened – the leukaemia, her decision about the transplant and the legal action which had been dropped – and thought nothing more of it.

But a couple of days later I left Hannah at home with a carer while I went to drop Oli, Lucy and Phoebe off at school and arrived home to find cars and vans parked all along the country lane where we lived. Driving slowly past the crowd, I saw people holding cameras and others talking into mobile phones. A van with a satellite dish was even parked on the side of the road, and as I pulled the car onto the drive and got out a woman rushed at me with a microphone.

'Mrs Jones?' she said, and I stared at her, unsure of what to say or do. 'Are you Mrs Jones? Hannah's mum?'

The group of reporters moved forward like a swarm as they pushed towards me. Cameras started clicking, microphones were switched on. Were they all here to find out about Hannah's holiday insurance?

'Are you Mrs Jones?' the woman asked again impatiently.

'Yes,' I said.

'I'd like to talk to you about Hannah's decision.'

'What do you mean?'

'The transplant.'

I didn't understand what she was talking about.

'We're here about Hannah,' another voice said as the cameras got closer. 'We want to talk about her decision to say no to a transplant – Hannah's right to die.'

It was the start of a media storm for which we could never have prepared. The story of Hannah's decision was covered by every newspaper and television station in the UK, as well as the world. Television stations and newspapers from Spain, Germany, Australia, Russia and France to Norway, Portugal, America, South Africa and New Zealand covered the story, and Hannah's choice sparked a furious debate about a child's ability to make such an important decision.

The phone rang every minute of every day, interview requests poured in and I allowed Hannah to do some because she was so excited at the thought of being filmed and photographed by newspapers and television. I also felt quietly proud that she could speak her mind so eloquently, and the coverage seemed like a tribute to her stoicism and bravery. If Hannah's decision inspired another parent to have the courage to make the right one for their child, even if it meant going against the collective wisdom, then she would make a mark on the world few children had the opportunity to create.

Soon letters were pouring through our door, some simply addressed to 'Hannah the girl with the poorly heart', written by ordinary people who had been moved by her bravery. On some days ten arrived, on others there were as many as eighty, and we ended up receiving more than 1,000. Hannah wanted to reply to them all, and on just one day we wrote 120 letters of thanks.

But I was unprepared for the storm of controversy her decision would create as journalists, commentators and the general public debated her decision in the pages of newspapers, on television and internet sites. Although there was mostly an upswell of support for Hannah's choice, there were those who didn't think she should have been able to make it, and while I tried to keep it from her Hannah had the internet and curiosity on her side. She also had to contend with the questions of sceptical journalists and soon picked up on what was being said. But instead of being upset she was angry, and I felt reassured by her strength of mind once again.

Negative reactions aside, though, the publicity did what I'd hoped it would and soon an anonymous company had agreed to put up the money for Hannah's insurance. Their kindness, and that of everyone who supported Caudwell Children, gave us a unique experience because the real world seemed another place when we flew to Disney World in December. We all forgot in that fairytale kingdom, even if it was for just a few moments as we stared at a firework show or stroked a dolphin. But for me perhaps the most memorable moment came as I stood with Hannah waiting for Phoebe to finish a ride.

'Excuse me?' I heard a voice say and turned to see a man smiling at us.

His accent sounded South African and he was smartly dressed, in his early fifties.

'I think you're the little girl I've seen on the news?' he said as he looked at Hannah.

She didn't seem sure of what to say and I wondered for a moment if I should usher her away from this stranger who seemed so keen to talk.

'I'm sorry to interrupt but I had to speak to you,' the man continued. 'I've read about your story and I just wanted to say that I think you're a brave girl. You should be able to do exactly what you want, Hannah, and I'm pleased that you are. Your story is an inspiration.'

The man smiled again before starting to turn away.

'I'll let you get back to your ride now,' he said. 'I'm sorry to barge in.'

I reached out to touch his arm. I wanted to say something, let him know how much his words had touched me.

'Thank you,' I said. 'Thank you so much.'

To know that a stranger from the other side of the world had read about Hannah and understood her choice meant more than I could say.

∾

We continued to collect memories: Hannah's eyes widening as she met Prince Charles at Clarence House, her smile as we sat down for Christmas lunch, her breath catching in cold winter air. More were created as 2009 got under way: Lucy and Hannah laughing as they sung along to CDs, the sound of Hannah's happy voice as she chatted to Simone about school, her excited face as she tumbled out of the car after a week in Cornwall over the Easter school holidays with Andrew, Oli, Lucy and Phoebe. I wrapped each happy moment up carefully in my mind, storing them away like precious family porcelain nestling in tissue paper, the mental history of our family life.

But however many memories I was given during the two precious years after Hannah left hospital having had the pacemaker, I still couldn't feel grateful when I began to realise that time might finally be running out. In May Hannah had a scan at Birmingham which showed her heart function was slightly lowered and I greedily wished that the world could stop turning and leave us where we were, for everything to stop so that we could be left for ever suspended in those happy memories. I'd always known this might happen but didn't feel ready for it.

I told myself that nothing was sure, maybe this was a temporary blip, maybe Hannah's heart function would increase again by the time we went back for another scan in three months. Although weaker, she was still up and about and looking forward to a trip we were making in a few days to a horse show that Lucy was competing at. Hannah was longing to come with us but I felt unsure about whether to allow her after the scan because we would be away for the weekend which would take a lot out of her. But as she excitedly prepared with Lucy, packing up the lorry and shouting orders at her sister, I knew that I couldn't bring myself to dash her hopes.

Just as I'd feared, though, the journey to the show exhausted Hannah, and she had to go straight to bed by the time we arrived. She and Lucy had planned to sleep together in the alcove above the driver's seat but she wasn't strong enough to get up the ladder to reach it. I thought of the day at the horse show just a few months before when she had climbed up to stow away. It seemed so far away as I settled her down to sleep on a camp bed, covered in blankets.

The rest of the weekend was the same – trying to keep things as normal as possible for Hannah, knowing I couldn't turn around and take her home because she would be outraged if I did, but sensing deep within me that something was changing. Hannah had had bad days before, but they were getting more frequent and took longer to recover from now. It was a week before she was out of bed again after the show and although Hannah got up as soon as she felt well enough – going up to London overnight with Andrew to visit the British Heart Foundation and celebrating Phoebe's birthday in early June – sadness filled me as I watched her. I was desperate to keep positive but knew that a day would come when Hannah's will was no longer enough to sustain her heart – and I feared it would be soon.

‑‑‑

'Would you like some oxygen?' I asked Hannah as she prepared to go to sleep.

'No,' she insisted.

'Why don't you just have it on for a while? I'll turn it off later when I go up to bed.'

'I'm fine, Mum. I don't want it. It's uncomfortable. I can't sleep with the line on. It hisses.'

It was six weeks since the horse show and Hannah had been getting slowly weaker. The changes were so small that someone who didn't know her well might hardly notice them. But I did. Each extra hour in bed, additional dose of anti-diuretics or anti-coagulants, told me that her heart was weakening.

'I really think you might feel better with some oxygen,' I said.

'I won't. I'll just go to sleep and tomorrow I'll be all right again. Please, Mum. I don't want it.'

I bent to kiss her and turn off her light, knowing that when she finally fell asleep I would creep back into her room and switch on the oxygen cylinder. Then I would push a mask as close to Hannah's face as I dared without waking her up and switch it off a few hours later so that she would never know what I had done. I wanted her to have the few moments of possible relief that the oxygen might give her even if she didn't.

The question of a transplant was hanging heavier in the air around us than it had for months. For so long it had seemed so far away, something that Hannah could almost forget as she revelled in all that she had achieved. But things were changing, and however much Hannah didn't want to acknowledge they were I felt sure that she understood what was happening.

I still felt afraid about all the risks a transplant held and what they might mean for Hannah. The longer she had been at home, the more important it had become to me that if she lost her fight she would do it peacefully in a place she loved. I felt afraid that if she had the operation she might reject the heart and die in hospital. The thought scared me more than anything. But another part of me understood why Hannah might change her mind now. Two years ago in hospital she had been too weak and afraid, too tired of being ill, to say yes. Now she had seen life again, had tasted all it had to offer and might feel ready to make a new decision.

I felt almost desperate, wanting to know what Hannah was thinking, sensing that the transplant was in her mind again, but afraid to push her and make her feel pressured to have one. She was still adamant every time it was mentioned but I knew she had spoken a little to a paediatric nurse who had started visiting again as her condition worsened to check her weight and medications. It wasn't until one morning in late June that she finally spoke to me as I sat on her bedroom floor while she rested and we watched television together.

'Mum?' she asked and I looked up at her. 'I have been thinking about the transplant.'

'What have you been thinking, Han?'

'About things like the medicines and how long I'd be in hospital afterwards.'

'Would you like to know more about that?'

'I think so.'

I stilled myself for a moment.

'I think I'd like to go and see the doctors at Great Ormond Street,' she said.

Hannah lay pale and quiet on the bed as I reached up to take her hand.

'OK, darling,' I replied softly, fear and relief welling up inside me.

The colours glared bright on the screen as I looked at it. Hannah and I were at Great Ormond Street and had earlier talked to a transplant nurse about exactly what the operation would entail if Hannah decided to have it. The nurse had told us about the surgery, the risks and recovery time, the follow-up appointments and drug regime that Hannah would be on for the rest of her life if she went ahead with the transplant. Now a consultant was giving her a heart scan and Hannah lay quietly on a bed as the probe was run over her chest.

I stared at the image of her heart.

The picture burned into me.

Blood rushed blue and red across the screen as the valves on the left side of her heart pumped weakly.

But the ones on the right were not moving at all.

Those valves were still.

I knew what I was seeing and it felt as if I was falling off a cliff and swooping towards the ground. I wondered if Hannah could see it too but she didn't say anything as she watched the screen, and when the scan was finished I pushed her out of the room in her wheelchair before stopping in the corridor.

'I just want to ask the doctor a couple of questions, Han,' I said. 'I won't be a minute.'

I had to be sure of what I'd seen before I decided what to tell Hannah, and so I left her with a nurse as I walked back to see the doctor, wanting to run but knowing I had to face the truth of whatever he was going to tell me.

'How bad is it?' I asked him quietly.

'Very,' he said. 'Hannah's heart is very, very weak. In fact the right side of it is not working at all.'

My breath caught in my throat.

'There is also a very significant area of clotting at the top of Hannah's heart which is pooling at the bottom of it. I'm afraid that one of those clots could break off at any moment.'

'What would happen if it did?'

'Hannah could go into arrhythmia because the beat of her heart would be affected, which might make her fall unconscious or cause her chest pain. The other possibility is that she could suffer a catastrophic stroke.'

I heard the words as if from far away and struggled to take them in. I hadn't prepared myself for news like this. So definite. So final. There was no chink of uncertainty any more. Hannah's health was no longer a question of opinion or possibility. The news was absolute. The right side of her heart had completely failed. I felt panicked, breathless almost, as I listened.

'How long does she have?' I asked eventually.

'It's her fourteenth birthday next week, isn't it?'

'Yes.'

'I can't say for sure that she will not see it, but I am certain she won't make her fifteenth.'

'But we've been told this before,' I said, desperate to make this all go away, fighting against the certainty in the doctor's voice, the memory of what I'd seen for myself on the screen.

'No one could be sure what the future held for Hannah when she last left hospital,' he told me. 'Her heart was weak but functioning and the pacemaker had also only just been put in. Nothing was certain.'

'But it is now?'

'I'm sorry, Mrs Jones, but yes.'

A thousand contradictions filled me – my mind clicking into practicalities like morphine and oxygen, anything to make sure that Hannah did not suffer – even as I wanted to run into the corridor and plead with her to have the transplant.

'If Hannah decides to go ahead with the transplant then we will need to know straight away,' the doctor said. 'You must also know that if she leaves it too long and her other organs begin to fail then she would not qualify for a new heart even if she changes her mind.'

There was nothing more to say. Hannah had to decide what she wanted because soon it might be too late. But I could not force her to make a quick decision or deny her this final say in her destiny, however afraid I felt. We had always believed in each other, and now we must again. Just as it always had been, this was Hannah's choice.

Hannah was walking out of her bedroom as I opened the door.

'Can I have a word with you, darling?' I asked, and she stopped.

It was the day after we'd been to Great Ormond Street and I had thought again and again about this conversation ever since we had travelled back from London. Hannah had been quiet in the car and so had I, both unable to speak of what hung heavy in the air between us. But now we must talk because she was leaving for a visit to Acorns tomorrow and the doctor's words were echoing in my mind. Time was running out.

As I walked to Hannah's bedroom I had remembered her lying on a hospital bed as blood spots burned red across her body so many years ago, the pink tears which had tracked down her face during the chemotherapy, her smile of wonder as she'd stared at the first tufts of downy hair growing back on her head.

Then I had pictured her face flushed with excitement as she got in from school, her delight when she had sat down to eat lunch with us all last Christmas, her quiet happiness about going up to the field with Lucy to see Mr Minty. These were the memories we must treasure now because they were all we had hoped for when Hannah had left hospital. But hope couldn't forge a path ahead for us any more, and I had to make sure she understood that she must decide what she wanted to do before it was too late.

'Can I talk to you, Han?' I asked.

She stopped what she was doing and turned towards me, her face pale and tired.

'I want to talk to you because your scan at Great Ormond Street was very bad,' I said softly.

Her gaze was steady.

'I know,' she replied.

I paused for a moment before speaking again, hating every word I was going to say but knowing I had to.

'The doctors think that if you don't have the transplant then you are probably going to die very soon. Your heart is very weak now and you need to decide what you want to do.'

Tears pricked bright in Hannah's eyes and I put my arms around her. I had to be strong, make sure she knew exactly what might happen, because I could not protect her from this anymore however much I wanted to.

'If you don't have a transplant then you will probably have your birthday next week but not your fifteenth,' I said, trying to keep my voice steady, bury the fear inside me so that she wouldn't hear it.

I felt afraid. Would Hannah think I was giving up on her? I had always said we'd prove the doctors wrong, but now I couldn't any more and I wanted her to understand why. Hannah must know the complete truth and I had to speak it. To make a choice, she had to know everything.

'I want you to understand how urgent this is, Han,' I said as I held on to her. 'That's why I'm telling you this.'

She was silent and I lowered my head next to hers.

'We can do whatever you want, Han, and if you decide that you still don't want the operation then you must know that I will make sure you don't feel any pain. I will always be with you. I will always be here. You will not be alone.'

Determination wrestled with fear on her face. As I looked at her, I wished harder than ever before that I could take her pain away.

'If this is too hard then Daddy and I can make the decision for you,' I said softly. 'You don't have to decide anything, Han, if you don't want to. Would you like to know what we would choose?'

She nodded.

Last night, Andrew and I had talked about the transplant and agreed what we would decide if Hannah asked us to. I had never spoken to her like this before but I could see she was struggling and wanted to help her carry the burden of the decision. She needed to know that if she wanted to say yes we would support her, but also understand that if she couldn't choose we could do it for her.

'Daddy and I think we would say yes to the operation.'

Neither of us moved.

'If you don't want it then that is absolutely fine, Hannah. You know that whatever you want is OK with us. You have said no before and you can say no again. We just want what is best for you, and that is whatever you are comfortable doing.'

She pulled away and looked up at me.

'I'm frightened,' she sobbed.

'What of, my darling?'

'Of asking you and Daddy and something going wrong because then you'd feel guilty, and I don't want that.'

I bent my head towards her.

'Hannah, you must never feel you can't ask us to decide,' I said. 'If you did then we would try our best to make the right decision and we couldn't feel guilty if we tried our best because that's all anyone can ever do.'

'Yes,' she said quietly.

'So that's what Daddy and I would do, and if you want us to help you decide then we can.'

'But I don't know what I want.'

She looked tired, as if the weight of the world was resting on her shoulders.

'Well, you don't have to decide tonight, do you?' I said softly. 'I want you to go to sleep now and think about this tomorrow.'

I knew I had to give her more time. But as Hannah settled down to sleep I knew that tomorrow might not come. We could not be sure of anything any more.

CHAPTER ELEVEN

The Gift of Life

❀

I can't stop thinking about the transplant. I've been at Acorns for four days, but when I'm lying on my bed or eating lunch or swimming or playing on Singstar it's there in my head all the time. I know it's in everyone else's too. The Chitty Chitty Bang Bang looks are really bad now.

We went to Great Ormond Street last Friday, and after years of going to scans I knew my own heart when it came up on the screen. I could see it wasn't working properly, but when Mum told me just how bad it was I couldn't help but wonder how I'm still here. I don't understand how I can do everything I'm doing when my heart is so bad. I know I've been getting more tired, but I've tried not to think about it and so I wished I had never gone to Great Ormond Street because I'd never have found out how bad things were.

But now I've got to make the decision. That's all there is to it. I know that if I don't have the transplant then I won't see fifteen. My fourteenth birthday is only five days away so it's only three hundred and seventy days until my fifteenth. There have been seven hundred and eighteen days since I left hospital, and that doesn't feel like long ago. So three hundred and seventy days doesn't seem like much time.

I don't want to have my fourteenth and then nothing.

I used to be sure, but now I'm in the middle.

It's hard.

I don't know what to do.

I feel too tired to think any more.

Mum and Dad have told me they can decide if I want them to, and I've nearly asked them loads of times. But I haven't because I still want to make my own decision. I know it would take the pressure off me if Mum and Dad chose, but they might feel guilty if I died after the transplant and I don't want them to live with that. I love them too much. They've got Oli, Lucy and Phoebe to look after so I don't want them to be sad if something happened to me after they had decided what to do. They've said they wouldn't, but even though they've promised me I still don't want to ask them.

Mum talked to me after we got back from Great Ormond Street and told me I wouldn't live long if I didn't have the transplant. That made me feel really sad but I still did not know what to do. Did I really want a massive operation? Could I promise to always take the pills I'd need to? The next day she brought me here and asked me again if I'd made up my mind. I told her I hadn't and she said that was fine and we'd talk about it when I got home. But I don't know how I'm going to choose, and I leave Acorns tomorrow. It's not a yes, it's not a no, it's a don't know. How do you work that out? Trying to decide between having a transplant and keeping going as I am is like being asked to pick between doing some really hard maths or running a marathon. I don't really want to do either one.

I wish things could be like they were.

How have I kept going when my heart is so weak?

The doctors say a transplant will only work if I really want it to and they won't do one unless I'm sure. I know I could die either way, but heaven doesn't scare me. When I think of it I see a place where you can do what you want and be with people you know who've gone before you. I'm not sure what it would look like, but if I had to guess then I'd say there would be a lot of grass and sky and people playing table tennis. I know that when I arrived in heaven I'd be fine and if I could I would send my mum a message to tell her that. I'd want her to know I was OK.

But I am scared of getting to heaven. Would it hurt? What if something went wrong with a transplant? I know some children do really well after them, but the doctors have told me it's not always like that, and I'd also have to take tablets for the rest of my life. What happens if I decide I don't want to one day? I've done that before. There have been days when I just couldn't take my pills, and if I had the transplant then I could never do that again.

But what if I don't have one?

I have no idea how I'll work this out.

My head feels fuzzy when I think about it.

I've been telling myself that I've been pretty determined before so I should be able to be again. The scan scared me, though, and I knew I couldn't think 'I'll prove you wrong' any more. I've been close to death's door three times and I'm still here. But I'm not sure what will happen now.

I've been really tired this week. I've tried doing things like going swimming or on the computer but I feel so tired that I don't even want to talk or watch TV a lot of the time. All I can do is lie down. I wasn't even sure I wanted to see Simone when she asked to come and visit me on Monday and I um-ed and ah-ed about it. But then she arrived and I was glad she had come because she brought flowers, chocolates, gum balls and giant strawberries. She also made me laugh when she told me about her mum putting salt in the crumble instead of sugar because her dad had changed the pots without telling her.

Then we did my favourite Acorns thing, which is going in the pool. I could not do much but it was great anyway and afterwards Simone and I had lunch before watching *Bride Wars* because I was feeling tired again. I didn't talk to Simone about what was going on, and she didn't ask. She knows I'd rather get on with it and she wants to make the best of it when she sees me, just like I do. She doesn't want to sit and ask questions all the time.

But Mum came to see me yesterday and we talked a bit. She asked me if I'd thought about the transplant but I didn't say too much because I was feeling really poorly. I had no energy and all I could do was lie on the sofa or in bed. I also had stomach pains and I felt scared when I went to bed last night because that's always the worst time. But Mum was with me, which made me feel better, and she sat with me so I got to sleep in the end.

I don't know what to do.

I can't decide.

At least I got my questions answered at Great Ormond Street. I wanted to know things like how long my recovery would be, how big my scar would be and what would happen after the operation. I also asked the transplant coordinator if there would ever be a time when it would be too late to change my mind, and she said yes. That really stuck in my head even though I didn't find out exactly when it would be. I'm glad I didn't ask that one.

But I know I don't have for ever.

I want to do everything I dream of doing.

Who doesn't?

What's on the other side?

These are the things that stop me from wanting a transplant:

- What happens if it goes wrong?
- What happens if I don't want to take pills for ever?
- What will Mum and Dad think if I decide yes? I'm worried they might think I've wanted it all along and haven't said.

The things that make me want to have one are:

- I will be well again if it goes OK.
- Lots of children have transplants and are fine.
- Not having one scares me as much as having one now.

Then when it's all running around my head I wonder if I really have a choice anyway. Maybe I just need to be more positive, think of the good things about having a transplant rather than the bad. When I said no before, I'd been in hospital and I was sick of it. But now I've been out of hospital for nearly two years and I've done so many great things which have reminded me of all there is left to do. Things are different now.

I want to have my Sweet Sixteen party, learn to drive and go on the ferry to Brittany with everyone. Mum speaks French so she could come, Dad could as well even though he can only speak German which won't be much use. But it would be good to have him there, and Oli, Lucy and Phoebe could come too. We could eat croissants and try some snails. I want to go on holiday and swim in the sea. I want to run in a field and dance to loud music. I want to see the world and visit all the places I've only read about in books. I want to be at home and play in the snow, go blackberry picking next autumn.

I want to see and do everything.

I used to think I could do it all without the transplant, and I did a lot. I proved everyone wrong, and I'm happy about that.

But it's not the same any more.

I don't want to die.

I want to live.

Hannah was quiet, just as she had been ever since I picked up her from Acorns four days ago. I knew she was close to making a decision about the transplant, but not yet, not quite yet.

'Maybe I'll have it,' she'd told me as we drove home from Acorns in the car.

'Would you like me to ring Great Ormond Street and tell them?' I'd asked her.

'No. I'm not completely sure.'

I longed to climb inside Hannah's head and find out exactly what she was thinking because then I might be able to help her more. Like any mother, I wanted to protect and comfort her, be part of her innermost thoughts. But what mother knows exactly what their thirteen-year-old is thinking? Very few, I suspect, and I had learned to allow Hannah to think, or not to think, to talk, or not to talk.

There was just one thing I wanted to allay her fears about. I did not want fear or ignorance to hold Hannah back from making this decision and was sure that the fact that a donated heart would once have belonged to someone else was playing on her mind.

'You know you won't change if you have a transplant,' I told her after she got back from Acorns.

Her face was guarded as I spoke.

'I know you've been thinking about it, Han, but it's your brain that makes you who you are, not your heart. It's your brain that gives you thoughts and feelings.'

'But what if I don't want the heart after I've had it?' she asked. 'What if I don't take my medicines and waste a heart that someone else needs?'

'I don't think you will if you decide it's what you want, Han. That's why you're thinking so hard. You want to be sure. And once you are, I don't think you'll change your mind.'

'No,' she said.

'And if you have the operation then I can't think of a little girl anyone would want to help more than you. When people decide to donate their hearts or their relatives do, it's to help someone who's very sick. I can't imagine a more worthy person than you – kind and good, strong and brave.'

But still Hannah had waited, and I knew the final hurdle which stood between her and a decision was her fourteenth birthday tomorrow. I was sure this was stopping her from speaking her mind and, however much I wanted to, I couldn't change the fact that details like birthdays and the size of her scar were important to Hannah. Those were the things she worried about, and she had missed so many birthdays over the years that they had become precious to her – unique days on which she could feel almost normal as she ate too much cake, opened presents and had fun just like her friends did. A day to forget.

Hannah's fifth and seventh birthdays had been spent in hospital after the leukaemia, she'd turned twelve on a high dependency unit after the heart failure and been ill in bed last year for the beginning of her teens. Each missed birthday stayed with her, and Hannah knew that from the moment she said yes to a transplant she might have to go back into hospital. She didn't want that, not quite yet, and nothing, not even the transplant, was going to stop her turning fourteen at home tomorrow.

And so I'd waited for four long days since bringing her home from Acorns, refusing to let my fears or impatience rush Hannah – forcing myself not to think of what was happening inside her, telling myself that time was precious but her peace of mind even more so. She had to be allowed to make this decision in her own time. She had to take the courage of her convictions into the operating theatre with her. I could not back Hannah into a corner because I feared she would say no if I did. She had been determined to make the most of the past few days and I was sure it was because she knew that once she said yes to a transplant things would be taken out of our hands. So she'd gone to a huge country gala with Andrew, Oli, Lucy and Phoebe, taking pictures of them all on rides, forcing herself to walk around in the sunshine before coming home exhausted. Her ability to cling onto every day amazed me and now she needed one final one that was hers.

But her birthday was almost here – we had planned her party, wrapped her presents, invited her friends and bought a cake. Hannah could finally be sure that she would celebrate as she wanted to, and I knew that I must talk to her again. Both of us were increasingly restless, finding it hard to sleep and unable to relax. When I'd checked on her in the night Hannah had been awake, and I'd sat with her until she fell asleep again.

Now I had to dare to push her just a little.

'I want to talk to you, Han,' I said as I sat down next to her. 'Because I think you've made up your mind.'

'Yes,' she said quietly.

One word which spoke a thousand.

'If you have decided about the transplant then I'm going to ask you to tell Great Ormond Street,' I said softly.

'I won't have to go back into hospital before tomorrow?'

'No, darling. We don't have to tell anyone except Great Ormond Street about your decision. No one else needs to know if you don't want them to.'

'OK.'

I slowly dialled the number to talk to Nadine, Great Ormond Street's transplant coordinator.

'Hello?' she said as she picked up the phone.

'Nadine?'

'Yes.'

'It's Kirsty here. I think Hannah wants to talk to you.'

I handed her the phone. She looked almost afraid for a moment, the weight of her decision pressing down on her. I held my breath as she began to speak.

'I've decided,' she said.

Her words were faltering and there was a pause before she spoke again.

'I want to go onto the transplant list. I want to have the operation.'

She finished speaking and passed the phone back to me. When the call was finished, I bent to hug her.

'I want to go on holiday and do my GCSEs,' Hannah told me.

'I know you do, darling,' I whispered. 'And I want you to as well.'

❧

Hannah lay back on the pillows in her bed. She was tired after her birthday party and needed to sleep now. Outside the sky was still light, the end of a warm summer's day, and I pulled the curtains closed to darken the room.

It had been a wonderful day. Hannah was as excited as she always was about birthday presents and had even had three birthday cakes after Grandma, a friend and I had all bought one. Earlier that afternoon we'd celebrated with her school mates Simone, Becki, Brigitta and Laura and Lindy's daughter Becky. Hannah had laughed with them and eaten cake, looked through a huge book full of photos and messages from school friends and teachers and even tried some tricks that a circus performer who'd come to the house had shown her – giggling as she twirled coloured ribbons on sticks or watched her friends try to stand on wobble boards. Grandma and Grandpa, Oli, Phoebe and Lucy had also been with us. It had been exactly the day that Hannah had wanted and I'd watched her smiling face knowing that I would hold onto the memory throughout everything that was to come.

The only thing she'd been anxious about after deciding to have the transplant was what other people would think.

'People change their minds about small things, and you've done it about a big one,' I told her. 'It's far braver to say you've changed your mind than be too scared to admit that you have.'

Now she seemed calm as she settled back in bed. In three days we would go to Great Ormond Street where tests would be done to decide if Hannah could go onto the transplant list. Although she had said yes, it was not certain that she would qualify for the operation because the doctors needed to check her other organs were healthy enough to cope with such major surgery. They also had to do complex blood typing to ensure her body would accept the heart because she had had so many transfusions in the past. If she did go on the transplant list, no one knew how long we would have to wait until a heart became available.

'Did you have a good day?' I asked Hannah as she sat up and I handed her some water to swallow her pills.

'The best,' she said.

'I'm glad.'

'Me too.'

'Mum?'

'Yes?'

'I love you.'

'I love you too, Han.'

My eyes opened wide. It was 3 a.m. I was finding it hard to sleep now, fearful that Hannah might not be strong enough to wait for a heart. It was less than a week since her birthday but her health had deteriorated even more. Each night now I went down to check her every hour and give her medicines to ease her pain or oxygen to help her breathing if she needed them.

I got out of bed and walked downstairs. A light glowed softly in Hannah's room as I walked in and saw her lying on the bed – her face was grey, her hands were clasped to her chest and her breathing was ragged. She looked afraid.

'Are you OK, Han?' I asked as I bent down to her.

'My chest hurts,' she gasped. 'It's like someone is sitting on me.'

'Don't worry, darling,' I said gently. 'I'm going to give you some medicine and then you'll feel better. Wait just a minute.'

Walking to the kitchen, I took aspirin and painkillers out of the cupboard. Panic threatened to overwhelm me. Was this it? Was Hannah dying? Not now. Please not now. Not when we'd come so far.

I helped her sit up as she gulped down the medicines and I gave her some oxygen before sitting down beside her bed.

'You're tired, Mummy,' she said.

'I'm fine, Han. You rest now.'

As the medicine kicked in and her pain eased, Hannah slipped back to sleep, and I sat with her. Just the two of us. Waiting for the dark hours of the night to slip slowly towards the light, another day. I wondered how this would end. I wanted Hannah to have the transplant now, wasn't sure I could bear to wait any more. I knew I had to let things happen in their own time, just as I always had, but this felt different. Hannah had decided. Once she had wanted to live without the operation and she had. Now she knew she couldn't carry on living without it.

The next morning, Hannah was taken into hospital where I was told her urea and creatinine levels were falling – her kidneys were beginning to fail and her blood pressure was low.

Time was running out.

Waiting.

Waiting.

Hannah's name is on the transplant list.

How long will it take?

Will she die before someone else does, someone whose heart might save her life?

Guilt and hope mix inside me.

How can I hope for a heart from someone who was loved just as Hannah is?

It is three weeks since Hannah's birthday and we've been in and out of hospital ever since. Her kidneys are getting worse and she is retaining more and more fluid. The doctors have increased her drugs and we've tried to go home. But now Hannah is back in hospital, too ill to be anywhere else. Her health is rapidly deteriorating.

There was a glimpse of good news last week: Hannah was on the transplant list, then another moment of hope a few days later when a heart became available. We got into an ambulance and started on the journey up to London before a phone call came to tell us that the heart was not suitable.

Hannah's face was stunned as the ambulance turned around.

How to keep her hope alive?

In the days that followed, Hannah made friends on the hospital ward with another little girl. Her name was Molly. She was having her appendix out.

They watched a DVD and chatted.

I talked to Hannah about the weather, what Oli, Lucy and Phoebe were doing at school, when Andrew would next come to visit.

Waiting.

Waiting.

I must keep Hannah strong, keep her hope alive.

But tonight I don't know if Hannah can wait any more. She is so weak now. Too tired to get out of bed or even talk much, she has been put back on Dobutamine to keep her fragile heart beating.

'I hope a heart comes tonight, Mummy,' she says as I settle her down to sleep.

'I know, darling,' I soothe. 'Let's pray that it does.'

Her blood pressure is dropping. The doctors have decided to space out her medications because her body is too weak to cope with them in large doses.

Down and down, her blood pressure is falling all the time.

It is 49/22. A healthy pressure is 120/60.

Please God.

Will she be too weak to survive the operation?

At midnight her consultant comes to see me. Hannah will have to be transferred to London in the morning. She needs life support. It's the only thing that will keep her alive now.

She lies sleeping.

Please.

Help.

Her.

The door opens and her consultant walks in.

'I have news,' she says and the world slows down. 'A heart has become available.'

My tears feel warm on my cheeks, just as they did on the day Hannah was born.

Will this be her second chance at life?

The blades of the RAF helicopter roared overhead. It was 4 a.m. – about two and a half hours since the call had come from Great Ormond Street. Hannah was too poorly to travel in an ambulance, and the helicopter was carrying a medical team from the Children's Acute Transport Service who had come to take her up to London. The helicopter had just landed outside Hereford Hospital, inching down into the available space just shy of the car park barriers. Trees bent in the helicopter's slipstream and fire engine headlights flooded the area in beams as the doors opened and people jumped out. Adrenalin pumped through my body as I looked at them, and a tiny part of me wondered if Hannah was really so ill – a mother's desperate denial about losing her child still pricking inside me even as I knew she lay dangerously sick upstairs.

As the CATS team went up to Hannah's room to prepare her to be moved, I packed our belongings. The new medics needed to change her Dobutamine line, check her vital statistics and make her as stable as possible for the journey. About an hour later we were ready to go and I said goodbye to the nurses who had looked after us so well over the past weeks. I'd felt close to them as we waited – all of us hoping that news would come soon – and I hugged them goodbye as we prepared to leave. Andrew was at home and would be on his way to London in the car as soon as his parents arrived to look after Oli, Lucy and Phoebe.

Hannah was stretchered outside and I followed close behind, watching her being lifted into the helicopter. Inside sat a navigator wearing a dark green helmet, ear defenders and a microphone, two pilots with helmets and visors and a winch man, who also wore a helmet and microphone.

But even with all this activity, Hannah had been too weak to be excited about the transplant or even frightened when I told her that a heart had become available.

'That's good,' she'd said, but nothing more.

Now she looked tiny as she lay on the stretcher with eight doctors and nurses sitting around her, their knees braced against the bed. Two drips stands stood beside her, she was connected to an oxygen mask and wore a helmet and ear defenders. My legs felt like jelly as I climbed into the helicopter and sat down before it took off into the dark sky. Was this the last journey that Hannah and I would make together? Was this the end of her life, or a new beginning?

About fifty minutes later we landed in Regent's Park where the sky had lightened. On this wet July dawn, joggers stared as the helicopter lowered to the ground and Hannah was put into an ambulance – the final stage of her journey to Great Ormond Street, a journey which had begun so many years before.

I watched the streets rush by as I sat beside Hannah.

'Nearly there, Han,' I said. 'Not too far now.'

She was quiet, self-contained within a shell of fear and anticipation as we arrived at Great Ormond Street, where we were taken up to the cardiac intensive care unit and told the surgeons were looking at the heart to make sure it was suitable. If it was, Hannah would go down for surgery within the hour, and as adrenalin pumped through her body, she became alert enough for us to play a board game half-heartedly as we waited.

When the transplant sister told us the heart was good, Hannah and I both knew it was time for her to go to theatre. It felt too quick. Andrew hadn't arrived yet because it was a three-and-a-half-hour drive to London and I knew he would be devastated to miss seeing Hannah. But there was nothing we could do, the doctors were ready and Hannah was put onto a stretcher and wheeled into the long hospital corridors. As I walked beside her I remembered the trips we'd made like these when she was a child. I wondered if she would be as frightened as she'd been back then when she was put to sleep today. I didn't want her to cry and scream, scrabble and fight to reach me as she was anaesthetised. I wanted her to be unafraid, to go into the operating theatre as peacefully as possible. She needed to take that certainty with her.

Hannah was pushed through double doors into a small square anaesthetic room where half a dozen doctors and nurses stood waiting for us. She looked so slight lying among them all and I talked to her softly as the anaesthetic was connected to one of her drip lines.

'I love you, Han,' I said over and over, a mantra for her to keep within as she fell asleep, a seed to plant deep inside as the surgeons worked to perform a miracle for her.

'I love you too,' she replied.

Her words rushed into me.

'I love you, Han.'

'I love you too.'

As the anaesthetic pulsed into her veins, I bent my head down towards hers.

'I want you to think of all we are going to do together,' I said as she looked into my eyes. 'When you wake up from this sleep, there will be so many things to do, my darling.'

Her eyes were calm as she looked at me.

'We are going to walk along the beach. Think of it, Han. Palm trees, white sand, water rushing onto the sand. That's where you are now. The air is warm, the sun is shining and you're walking into the sea. The blue, blue sea ...'

Hannah smiled lazily as she drifted into unconsciousness.

'And when you are home, we will watch Oli play football, go to see the horses with Lucy, go for walks along the lane ...'

I looked at her face.

She was sleeping now, peaceful. She was finally ready. She had made her choice.

CHAPTER TWELVE

A New Beginning

The sunshine was the lazy yellow of early autumn as Hannah and I walked along the lane towards the fields.

'There's one,' I said, and pointed to the hedgerow.

She took a step towards the brambles and carefully pulled a blackberry from a mass of tiny thorns.

'No good,' she said as she touched it. 'Too small. Hasn't had enough rain.'

She peered deeper into the hedge.

'That one looks better.'

She pulled the blackberry from the bush and popped it into her mouth.

'I was right!' she said, and giggled.

We walked on slowly in silence for a few moments as Hannah stopped now and again to pull more blackberries from the bushes. The sun was warm today. It had dried patches of mud to a thin crust on the road, and all around us the colours of early autumn were seeping across the country-side. Deep red, acid green, hot flashes of pink from the last remaining wild flowers, the creamy white of Old Man's Beard which littered the hedgerows.

'What time do we have to leave tomorrow?' Hannah asked.

'Very early, about 6.30, so you're going to have to go to bed in good time tonight.'

'OK.'

We were going to London for one of the weekly check-ups Hannah had been having since leaving Great Ormond Street. After tomorrow's we hoped to go just once a fortnight because the doctors were pleased with her progress.

It was two months since Hannah had come home, and while she remembered only snatches of being in hospital, memories of the eleven days she'd spent in intensive care after her transplant were still fresh inside me. The surgeons had been unable to close her chest at first because the cavity wasn't big enough to cope with a healthy heart. Hannah had been unconscious for ten days until the wound had finally been sewn up and every minute that she lay with her chest open was a minute too long for me because the risk of infection was so high.

Sealed in a room in intensive care, Andrew and I had had to put on gowns and aprons in an antechamber before opening the door to Hannah's room which shut with a hiss behind us to preserve the sterile environment. Computers stood around her bed and she lay in a pool of light hooked up to ventilators and other machines. There had been other problems too: Hannah's blood pressure was uneven, her kidneys still weak and she had not ingested her liquid feed properly.

But the doctors had always seemed pleased with her progress, and one had even told us how well she looked when her chest was still open. I could only wonder at what these surgeons had seen to make them so brave.

After her chest was finally closed, Hannah had begun to wake up again, and I was thankful that she did not remember those awful days in intensive care. Her memories only began after she'd been transferred to a ward for the final nine days of her stay, and she'd started to move and eat, talk and even laugh. I knew she was feeling better on the morning that she asked for a croissant and agreed to a game of Scrabble. Her hands were shaking too much for her to put the letters in place so I'd done it for her, quietly rejoicing in our first glimpse of normality.

On our final day before going home Hannah's surgeon had come to see us and I had thanked him for all he had done, knowing that words were almost useless in expressing our gratitude for the dedication and excellence of the team at Great Ormond Street. After that we'd taken Hannah home, and although she had been tearful and weak initially, her body and emotions drained by all that had happened in such a short space of time, she continued to get stronger.

Once again we measured our days by the most ordinary of things: Hannah getting out of bed and eating, sleeping well at night, feeling strong enough to go with Andrew for a short trip to the supermarket, walking 100 metres down the road with me to visit a friend who told us about her holiday to France as we sat in late afternoon sunshine.

The doctors had told us she would need three months at home before she could go back to school, and during that time we had to be careful about going to restaurants, cinemas or anywhere crowded with people who might pass an infection on to Hannah. So we had spent the time quietly at home, where her spirit gradually bubbled up inside her again as she did a little more each day. As Hannah realised she was growing stronger, her excitement and happiness about what she had to look forward to increased, and seeing her smile again was almost more than I had dared wish for.

'Mum?' she said as we reached the field where the horses were waiting for us.

She stood beside me as we got to the gate. Her cheeks were pink, her eyes were bright.

'Yes, Han?'

'Can we make blackberry jam when we get home?'

'Of course.'

'And then can I put on the *Mamma Mia!* soundtrack really loud?'

'Maybe, Han.'

'Go on.'

'We'll see.'

She giggled as she stood beside me and I took her hand as we walked into the field. The green grass stretched ahead of us, the sky was blue overhead and I felt inexpressibly thankful for this day.

Phoebe drew me a picture recently and I absentmindedly put it down as I rushed around. But when I got into bed that evening I made myself study it – the eyes, the hair, the lopsided smile on the face of a stick person – and it reminded me that I must never forget all that Hannah has taught me. To take notice of the tiny details of my children's lives, to stop and appreciate them, to see who they are and love them for it.

Our life is already changing – when Hannah walked a few hundred metres from the car to a ward on Hereford Hospital for a blood pressure check it felt like a hundred miles – and I am slowly learning to trust that it has. But it's a slow process and one that will take me some time, I think. The most critical period for organ rejection is during the first six months after transplant, and although the children are desperate for us to book a holiday next summer I can't yet quite bring myself to go from living from minute to minute to planning a trip nine months away. In the New Year I'll sit down, make a booking and allow myself to believe.

But I know that even as Hannah becomes stronger and our life slips back into a normal pattern I will guard against falling into the trap of constantly looking forward and forgetting today. I always want to honour the journey we have made because it taught me to live a life that is not as ferociously busy as so many people's. I don't want to run through days, weeks and months so fast that I don't have time to see them properly.

It wasn't always this way. Before Hannah first fell ill I was caught up in the business of life and suspect I might have wasted a little of its joy if it hadn't been for her. But she showed me a different path, and I hope I have given my children much of what I dream of for them – love and laughter, rules and freedom in equal measure. Most of all, I have tried to pass on what I have learned and teach them to enjoy every day for what it is.

When I think of Hannah, I think that she is three miracles rolled into one: first, she was conceived when I'd almost given up hope of becoming a mother; second, she survived leukaemia; and third, she is alive today. But maybe she is just one miracle, stronger than any of the other three because it's not about the body but the soul. Hannah has taught me more about life than I ever knew I had to learn and shown me things I did not know I had not seen. Our journey took us to some of the darkest places a parent or child can know and there were times when we all wondered if we'd chosen the right fork in the road. But it also took us into the light, to places we never expected to find where we learned a great deal. For that I will always thank Hannah, and her courage, determination and sheer love of life have shown me that it can be fully lived without necessarily being long.

It is one of the hardest things to remember when you fear your child is losing its battle against illness, and I have never forgotten a mother I once met who told me she could never forgive herself if she didn't do everything possible to save her child, try every treatment, however tiny the chance it might work. I understood her desperation and respected her choice. But I have learned that it is also possible to make a different one – enjoy your child and accept that lives sometimes have limits, however painful they are. You must have peace inside you to give to a sick child, and that is what I wanted for Hannah – the knowledge that I was on her side for right or wrong because knowing that I would always respect and defend her wishes made her feel safe. I believe it was the right thing for her.

Now I look forward to our future together and feel grateful every day to the person or family who gave Hannah this gift. They will never know our joy, but I will honour it by teaching my children as best I can. It is Hannah who has shown us to have a life of colour instead of grey, and that is all I want to give her in return. Hannah knows what colour her rainbow is, and I will continue allowing her to live it. It is the most that any mother can ask.

❀

Do you know that I'll never be able to eat grapefruit again? It interferes with an anti-rejection drug called tacrolimus that I'll have to take for the rest of my life, so don't give me a grapefruit and soda to drink if I ever meet you. That's just one of the things I can't eat now, and there are others. Sushi is one, but I'm not bothered about it because I don't want to eat raw fish. There are also things like cheeses and salami though that I'd like to eat but can't because they might make me sick, which wouldn't be good for my medication. That's the only bad bit about having a transplant – and the fact that I'll have to do PE when I get back to school.

But other than that, having a new heart is brilliant because I've got so much energy I don't know what to do with myself. My scar is not too bad, and no one can see it if I wear a top with a high neck. There are more important things to worry about anyway. When I first got home I couldn't tie up the laces on my trainers because it made me dizzy to bend down or walk more than a couple of minutes before I got tired. That worried me, and I wondered if the transplant had worked properly. But then

I got stronger and stopped watching the DVDs that everyone had given me. I just wanted to be up and about as soon as I could because I'd spent too much time lying in bed.

Now I can walk to see the ponies who are quite far down the road and I've even been to school for a few hours. I had to rest when I got home but I was fine again really quickly, which was great. These are the other things I've done: been to watch Oli play football, out for pizza, had Simone to stay, gone shopping and visited my Grandma and Granddad. But that's nothing compared to what I'm planning to do: go to the theatre, learn to swim better because I never had enough energy to get very far before, go to my friend Molly's Halloween party and stay with Simone at her house. I'm also going to a Christmas party that a friend of Grandma and Granddad's has in a barn every year, and next summer we're all going to Spain. How cool will that be? I can't wait to see Phoebe running in and out of the sea and jump in the pool with Lucy.

I think she's happy that we can do more stuff together now, and we've decided that we want an Xbox or a Wii. Mum says she doesn't mind if we get the money ourselves, so we've collected up all our old toys, books and DVDs which we're going to sell at a car boot sale this weekend. Dad has helped us by looking in the garage for things to sell, so we might let him have a go on whatever we buy, but we won't let Oli because he hasn't done anything.

After I had the transplant I met a man called Matthew who had one when he was nineteen. He was really nice and he even plays rugby now. I don't think I want to do that because I'm not sure I'd like running. I've never done it, but maybe I'll have to try it when I do gym at school. I can't wait to go to St Mary's every day again. At the moment my hospital tutor comes to see me for an hour a day, but things will be just like they were before when I get back to school.

The only thing that will have changed is the fact that I've gone off *High School Musical* because I've realised that everything is perfect in it and life just isn't like that. So now *Mamma Mia!* is my total favourite and I love it when Sophie says she's not going to get married at the end. She wants to see the world instead and that's what I'd like to do. I've also decided that I don't want to be a fashion designer or like Cheryl Cole any more. I want to be a vet or a singer instead.

Taking my pills now isn't too bad because I can have ten in one go. Did you know that? I can put them all in and swallow. When I was little I didn't even need water to do it, although I do now. That was one of the things which stopped me having the transplant before, and although I always knew I could change my mind I didn't want to. It was annoying when Mum kept checking up about it, and other people asked as well. I was sure I wasn't ready.

But then I began to get ill, and what helped me change my mind was the fact that I'd had good years after coming out of hospital. When I was first asked about the transplant I was really sick and just wanted to go home. Sometimes you can't listen to doctors and have to go with what you want whatever anyone else thinks. If I'd had the transplant when I was first asked about it I'd have been unhappy, and that wouldn't have been right.

But then I had good years and wanted to have more of them so I felt happy when I decided to say yes. I talked to my doctor at Great Ormond Street about it when I went for my last check-up and he said I just needed to think more, and he was right. I wanted to live when I said no and I wanted to live when I said yes.

That's what everyone got wrong when the newspapers started writing about me, and although most people were kind some weren't.

'I fear for Hannah's life,' one person wrote on a website. 'I fear she is too young and has made the wrong decision by refusing a heart transplant she obviously needs.'

It made me angry to read that because the person had judged me, and that's wrong. No one knows anyone else's life like they do, and I was young but I'd seen things most adults hadn't. Anyway, the person who wrote on the website didn't understand the most important thing: my decision about the transplant wasn't about dying. It was about living. And that's the same reason why I decided to have it.

I was scared, though, when it actually happened, and I never wanted the helicopter ride to London to end. Everything seemed to be happening so quickly, and although I knew that one girl had waited just thirty-six hours for a new heart I'd also been told another boy had had to wait a year. But it was too late to change my mind, and deep down I was sure. I feel thankful that someone gave me a new heart because I don't know where I'd be without it. That person saved my life, and what bigger thing can anyone do?

So now I'm going to keep getting better and be normal again. But when I am, I won't forget being ill because this is what I've learned:

- Try not to be down every day or think your life is worse than anyone else's.
- Make yourself do something you've never done before.
- Prove someone wrong.
- Get good grades in school so you can get a good job and buy nice things.
- Think about people worse off than you.
- Enjoy what you've got.
- Love your family and friends.
- Break a rule but not the law.
- Be brave.

That's it really. I just want to keep on getting better and do all the things I've thought about for so long.

So I suppose there's just one other thing to say. But really, it's the most important thing of all.

Watch out, world ...

I'M COMING TO GET YOU!

Acknowledgements

Our most grateful thanks must go to Dr Simon Meyrick at Hereford County Hospital, and our GP, Dr Andrew Knight, because without their care and knowledge Hannah would not be here today. Thanks to the rest of the team at Hereford County Hospital and those who got out of bed on the night of Hannah's transplant to help one child. They include the RAF, the CATS team, all at Great Ormond Street and Hereford firemen. Our thoughts, love and prayers go to the families who donate organs when they lose their loved ones and give the gift of life to another. Yours is an act of selflessness that must never be underestimated. Thank you Di, Winnie, Jess and Tina for their support with our horses even though Di lost her husband Ken during this time, and Lindy Boucott, who deserves a special mention for sitting with me night after night making the long dark hours bearable. She is a true friend. To everyone at Acorns, thank you for giving Hannah a home from home where she feels safe and happy. Thanks to Grandma and Grandad. And finally, lots of love to Oli, Lucy and Phoebe for trying hard to be so good and giving Hannah and me so many smiles over the past few years. Andrew, you were a constant and reassuring presence throughout everything. Thank you.